MAKING
FATS & OILS
WORK FOR YOU

A Consumer's Guide For A Healthier Life

LEWIS HARRISON

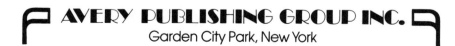
AVERY PUBLISHING GROUP INC.
Garden City Park, New York

The medical and health procedures in this book are based on the training, personal experiences, and research of the author. Because each person and situation is unique, the publisher urges the reader to check with a qualified health professional before using any procedure where there is any question regarding its appropriateness.

The publisher does not advocate the use of any particular diet and exercise program, but believes the information presented in this book should be available to the public.

Because there is always some risk involved, the author and publisher are not responsible for any adverse effects or consequences resulting from any of the suggestions, preparations, or procedures in this book. Please do not use the book if you are unwilling to assume the risk. Feel free to consult a physician or other qualified health professional.

Cover designers: Rudy Shur and Martin Hochberg
Cover photographer: Murray Alcosser
In-house editor: Cynthia J. Eriksen
Typesetters: Straight Creek Company, Denver, Colorado

Library of Congress Cataloging-in-Publication Data

Harrison, Lewis.
      Making fats & oils work for you / Lewis Harrison.
            p. cm.
      Includes bibliographical references (p.) and index.
      ISBN 0-89529-436-2
      1. Lipids in human nutrition—Popular works. 2. Consumer
      education. I. Title. II. Title: Making fats and oils work for you.
      QP751.H36 1990   90-658
      613.2'8—dc20   CIP

Printed in the United States of America

10 9 8 7 6 5 4 3 2 1

MAKING
FATS & OILS
WORK FOR YOU

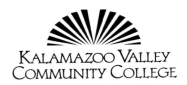

Contents

To Maharaj Charan Singh for his guiding light.

Acknowledgments

I would like to thank Joan and Lydia Wilen and Sid Jainchill for their kindness and openness beyond the call of duty. I am deeply indebted to Tanya, my love, for creating the space to research important material. My mother Dorothy's research efforts and wisdom were invaluable to me. I am also grateful to Vincent Collura for starting the project and to Marty Kalmanson, Marlene Goldstein, Mark Becker, and Dr. Daniel Wiener for supporting me when the hurricanes hit.

Preface

Fats and oils. Every day there is another report, study, or viewpoint presented about them. One day we are told that cholesterol is a killer, and the next day we are told that there are good and bad types of cholesterol. It is not difficult to understand why there is so much confusion about them. Just as people were beginning to think that they could make sense of it all, controversy over the effects of oat bran arose. Some scientists claimed that including oat bran in the diet could lower cholesterol, while others said that it was all commercial hype.

For these reasons, when the opportunity arose for me to write *Making Fats and Oils Work for You*, I was very excited. The task of clarifying the misconceptions that people have about fats and oils seemed like a worthy endeavor. This book is the result of my desire to convey accurate and helpful information about fats and oils in the diet.

Nutrition is an ever-changing science, and an in-depth discussion of nutrition, especially concerning fats and oils, could easily become technical. Although there is certainly no shortage of material written on fats and oils, I felt there was a need to write a book that could explain how fats and oils work in the body in laymen's terms, and to guide you, the reader, into using fats and oils wisely. Fats and oils should be included as part of a well-balanced nutritional program. There are many ways that fats and oils can be used for good health; hopefully, this guide will help you discover them. The key to reducing the dangers of fats while obtaining their benefits is to include them in your diet in the proper amounts and to avoid using them improperly.

The text is organized in a manner that, I feel, will make the information more accessible. Our use of fats and oils over more than 4,000 years has certainly changed. Chapter 1 gives you some basic background information on fats and oils, and discusses the changes that have occurred in the way we manufacture oil. It highlights the differences in flavor and nutritional value between traditional and mass-produced oils that exist due to the method of oil extraction used.

If you think that fats and oils have only negative effects on the body, you need to refer to Chapter 2, which explains how this nutrient is essential for certain body functions. Deficiencies in fats and oils can lead to numerous symptoms and poor health. Health problems arise from consumption of fats and oils only when the diet contains too much fat, or when it is obtained from poor food sources. Because obesity is one of the greatest health problems facing Americans today, Chapter 3 has been devoted to reducing fat in the diet.

Although dietary fat can be dangerous in excessive amounts, there are certain fats and oils that have beneficial effects. The therapeutic uses of various oils are discussed in Chapter 4. Most of us are well aware of the dangers of fats and oils. In the wrong amounts, they are a threat to good health. In Chapter 5, the health problems that can result from a diet high in fat are explored, and suggestions on how to reduce these risks are offered.

Chapters 6 and 7 are designed with the consumer in mind. First, Chapter 6 explains the advantages and disadvantages of using a particular oil with regard to its nutritional value, shelf life, and flavor. This section also offers tips on how to prevent oils from becoming rancid. Finally, Chapter 7 attempts to clear up misconceptions regarding food labels and advertisements, fat content, and the nutritional differences between butter and margarine and various other food products. It gives you helpful suggestions on reading labels for fat content. Appendices are also provided for easy reference, listing the fat and cholesterol content of different foods.

As you apply the information presented in *Making Fats and Oils Work for You*, you may find that this entire area of knowledge falls somewhere between the realms of culinary art and culinary science. By applying the information within, you will be able to make clearer and more educated decisions about your personal health and about the health of those who are close to you.

Introduction

Every day we are presented with confusing advertisements extolling the benefits or pointing out the negative effects of fats and oils. Among the many advertisements used to promote various food products, you may have seen or heard those claiming that the product is "high in polyunsaturates" or "low in fat," contains "no cholesterol," or contains "omega-3 fatty acids." Food companies try to persuade consumers to buy their products with statements such as "butter is better," "real people eat meat," and "cream cheese has half the calories of butter." There is a constant onslaught of conflicting points concerning every food from prepared meat to salad dressing. There is probably no nutrient that fills the public consciousness as much as fats and oils and no nutrient that has as many myths and controversies associated with it. Just think of all the different things you have heard or been told about cholesterol and about the relative nutritional values of butter and margarine, the health benefits of fish oils, and the dangers of beef fat. For years people have heard about the dangers of cholesterol, but now we know that there are different types of cholesterol—high-density lipoproteins and low-density lipoproteins, with the first being good for you and the second being bad. The confusing advertisements that we see extolling the fact that vegetable oil "contains no cholesterol" do not differentiate between the various types of cholesterol and the ways in which certain types of cholesterol are important for good health.

As valued commodities fats and oils have had a major impact on the history of the world through trade, wars, industrial developments, and modern food processing.

With the rise of consciousness about the dangers of certain types of cholesterol, followed by concern about triglycerides in the 1960s and 1970s, a campaign was mounted to bring people into the new fold: get rid of fats in your diet! Much was written and published to this end. Although the importance of fats and oils in the human diet has long been known, the emphasis here is on the level of *consciousness* that exists or doesn't exist on a wide scale. The truth is that oils and fats in precisely determined ratios are one of the indispensable constituents for human life. In order to maintain health, they cannot be reduced below the level needed to maintain that ratio. Yet much of the advice given was to cut down indiscriminately on our consumption of "fats." With so much new information available and the media maligning all types of fats and oils, there is a need for you to become informed about the true nature of these important nutrients and which types and how much of each type are required for good health.

There certainly is no shortage of scientific information concerning fats and oils. Because of the attention given them by hundreds of articles, documented clinical information, and scientific journals with their reports on disease, health, weight loss, and special cultural traditions, fats and oils are clearly in the public consciousness. The lack of knowledge concerning the importance of healthy fats and oils, however, can contribute to many health problems. Deficiencies of essential fatty acids can lead to many symptoms including heart abnormalities, fatigue, susceptibility to infection, dry hair and skin, eczema, allergies, acne, varicose veins, and kidney malfunctions. These disorders could all be prevented with as little as two daily tablespoons of the appropriate vegetable oil. This is one of many helpful hints that this book has to offer you.

Although most books on nutrition have small sections discussing fats, there is seldom any in-depth presentation of their essential qualities, and, more often than not, there is nothing more than a few passing comments concerning the dangers of fats, the rich taste that they add to foods, and the warmth and energy that they supply the body in winter.

This book is the result of a sincere wish to present you with helpful information about the role of fats and oils in the diet. By familiarizing yourself with the information provided in this book and by making use of it, you will be able to bring your health to a new level of excellence.

Regardless of your ethnic background, how fat or thin you are, or how tall or short, you are composed of ingredients that come from food. Studies in the last few years indicate that your mental health, moods, abilities, and attitudes are greatly affected by what you eat and how you prepare it. Although there is much information about nutrition available, much of it can be complex and confusing. Nature is truly a thing of beauty, and the simple act of eating and the body processes that are involved in utilizing food reflect this beauty on every level. When you eat a food, the grinding of your teeth and a chain of chemical processes all work to break down each mouthful into the basic elements that are essential for life: fats, starches, proteins, fiber, vitamins, minerals, and water. All of these enable your body to function and grow. When you take in more energy-producing nutrients than you use, your body stores them as fat. When people speak of fat, they are generally referring to some type of food that tastes great, but is low in nutritional value and high in calories.

Many people are not even sure what fats are or how they are different from oils. Fats and oils are complex compounds. They occur in various forms in plants and animals, and in tissue, blood, and cells. Because they are composed of various fatty acids, fats and oils do not all have the same nutritional value. Some are essential to health, while others may contribute to disease. It is the pleasing taste and texture that fats and oils give to food, their availability in so many forms, and their wide use in food preparation that have led to an excessive consumption of them.

Some people think that the body requires some nutrients like protein more than others, such as fats or carbohydrates, to maintain good health. No single nutrient is either more or less important than any other. Each is necessary for the health of all cells. What you should be concerned about are the amounts and sources of these nutrients.

Although Americans have been urged for years to reduce the amount of fat in their diets, particularly animal fat, this does not change the nutritional importance of fats and oils. Instead, it really emphasizes the importance of understanding the body's requirements for specific fats and oils, as well as the nutritional differences between the various kinds. If you do not understand how and why fats and oils are important, you can truly harm your health.

The purpose of this book, then, is to give you, the reader, a clear sense of how fats and oils affect all of our lives. By addressing the fundamental issues, this book may help you find ways of dealing with health problems that may be the result of faulty nutrition and conditioning. It explores the ways that fats and oils can be used to heal, and discusses the role that they play in cerebrovascular disease, heart disease, hypertension, diabetes, gout, and cancer. It is not my purpose to tell you what to do, or to teach you what and what not to eat; however, practical suggestions are offered that you can easily apply to your daily nutritional program. This is not a weight-loss book, nor is it an inquiry into the ways in which to create a fat-free diet. The intent of this book is to present clear and concise information that will help you understand the importance of fats and oils in good nutrition. It is my desire to present this information in a way that is less complex than a technical encyclopedia, which includes all scientific studies, footnotes, and present knowledge concerning fats and oils, but more in depth than what is generally found in books on basic nutrition. I want to offer you sufficient scientific information to assist you in making more intelligent dietary decisions. By helping you understand how fats are used commercially in food production and their effects on health and disease, I hope to enable you to decrease your chances of disease and promote good health.

There are many ways that this book can be used: as a general interest work to stimulate and enrich your appreciation of the history of fats and oils in the everyday lives of different people and their use in different cultures; as bedside reading to improve your health; as a reference text; or as a nutritional handbook. However you use it, you will find many applications to daily life.

By applying logic and reason to the information presented in this book, you will be able to uncover some of the secrets of nature, and surmise why certain foods are healthy for you and why others aren't.

Fats and oils can work for you. More than anything else, this is a book on obtaining and maintaining good health through the educated use of fats and oils. You will learn how to use them to promote vitality, fend off diseases, and extend your life. By applying the recommendations given, you will learn how to increase good fats by using foods that are high in them, while reducing bad fats and their food sources from your diet. We have been led to believe that cholesterol kills. This book will tell you what you need to know about cholesterol and its relationship to fats and oils and how to control it. Here's to good health through fats and oils.

1
History of
Fats and Oils

Every day we are bombarded with new bits of information on fats and fat-related subjects. We have been told that eating such-and-such a breakfast cereal is the "right thing to do" because it lowers cholesterol, that a particular oil is "high in polyunsaturates," that a burger has been "flame-broiled, not fried," and so on. It seems that when it comes to the topic of food, there is not much that one hears without some mention of fats and oils.

Although many people often assume that fat is a single substance, the accepted definition of fats or lipids generally includes a variety of organic substances. These can include oils, waxes, fats, and other related substances. What these all have in common is that they are greasy to the touch, will not dissolve in water, and will dissolve in ether or alcohol. Fats are commonly called lipids by both doctors and nutritionists.

A chemist would require greater specificity in his definition of a fat than the one offered above in order to be more accurate. A chemist knows that all fats belong to the class of organic compounds generally known as lipids. These lipids are composed of the same structural elements: carbon, hydrogen, and oxygen. Certain types of substances have the same general combination of carbon, hydrogen, and oxygen. These are known as fatty acids. What surprises many people is that carbohydrates are also composed of carbon, hydrogen, and oxygen. The primary difference separating fats from carbohydrates is the relatively higher hydrogen content of the fats. This hydrogen factor is what creates the substantial differences both in the way your body uses fats and carbohydrates and in their respective nutritional values. It is the relative hydrogen content of the fat that determines whether it is solid or liquid at room temperature.

THE FUNCTION OF FATS

Fats play many roles in the body, affecting the chemistry of the body as well as structurally protecting the vital organs. There are few body processes that do *not* involve fats on some level. Basically, fats serve three primary functions:

1.   They are a concentrated source of energy.
2.   They are a source of essential nutrients called *essential fatty acids.*
3.   They are essential for the transportation and absorption of fat-soluble vitamins A, D, E, and K in the body.

   Throughout this book fats will be referred to as polyunsaturated, unsaturated, monounsaturated, or saturated. These are all chemical terms used to refer to the way hydrogen is carried in the fatty-acid molecule. Most fats are not one type or the other, but are actually a combination of both unsaturated and saturated fatty acids. All of the various substances known as food fats can be divided into two categories: fats and oils. Let's take a look at the essential difference between these two substances.

THE DIFFERENCE BETWEEN FATS AND OILS

Why are some food fats classified as fats, while others are classified as oils? The level of saturation of the food fat will technically determine in which of the two categories it most appropriately fits, but the difference is not hard to point out, even to the untrained eye. Lipids that are liquid at room temperature, such as olive oil, are called oils, while those that are solid at room temperature, like lard and butter, are called fats. Many foods contain a combination of fats and oils.

Oil manufacturing has been in practice for more than four thousand years. Since this practice began, increased use of oils has led to changes in the ways we manufacture oils. As you read about how modern methods have been able to increase the amount of oil that can be extracted from seeds, increase an oil's shelf life, and decrease manufacturing costs, keep in mind the trade-offs that have been made in the aroma, flavor, and nutritional value of the oil.

THE HISTORY OF OIL MANUFACTURING

All of the various vegetable oils that you use come from the seed-bearing fruits of flowering plants. Many believe that the sesame seed was the first source of extracted oil. Records indicate that over four thousand years ago, the Assyrians and Chinese processed oil by roasting the seeds and finely grinding them with a mortar. They would then wait for the freed oil to rise in the bowl. Although sesame seeds are as much as 63 percent oil, these ancients would be lucky to get even one-fourth of that amount. The poor return on this process naturally led to the search for more effective ways of extracting oil.

Even up to the Second World War, much of the oil used was extracted at home. Any oil manufacturing that was done on a commercial level was primarily a small cottage industry. These small companies used slow, small cool-running presses to extract the oil. Fresh flax oil would be delivered weekly in 100 milliliter bottles much the same as eggs and milk were brought. Flax oil was used for its nutritional value and nutty flavor and medicinally.

The extraction of oil at home and by small companies began to fade in the 1920s. Huge oil-producing companies began to develop. These firms planted vast amounts of oil-producing seeds. These seeds were processed through huge presses designed to run twenty-four hours a day and capable of pressing over 100 tons of oil seeds a day. Pesticides and synthetic fertilizers came into play, greatly increasing crop yields. When automation reduced the cost of processing, the price of the oil also dropped.

New, more efficient processes for seed preparation and extraction were developed, and processing techniques that had never been used in oil manufacturing began to dominate the industry. Oils that had previously enjoyed a rich aroma and flavor but a limited shelf life were now refined, bleached, deodorized, and chemically preserved to increase shelf life. The small oil-producing companies all but disappeared as a result of the onslaught of low-cost, mass-produced oil. Oils like flax also disappeared since they were too unstable due to their nutritional "impurities" and likely to spoil. Interestingly, the two "impurities" that caused the instability of flax oil were linoleic and linolenic acids, two essential fatty acids that are probably the most valuable nutritional sources of fats and oils. Flax was thus replaced by oils having a greater shelf life and stability but a much lower nutritional value. Flaxseed oil is still used commercially in the manufacture of paint. When you boil flaxseed oil and add lead to it, linseed oil results. This oil takes on a "drying" quality that is very important to paints.

Most oils that you find on store shelves have been extracted either by a pressure process or by the use of solvents. The flavor and nutritional value of the oil will vary according to the method of extraction used.

The Pressure Process

In the pressure process the oil-bearing material is ground or flaked, and is then fed into a large cylinder with a wide worm shaft that revolves inside. The shaft, which resembles a large screw, presses the oil-bearing material against the walls of the cylinder and a big back plate. The oil is then expelled through the slots in the cylinder. Oils manufactured using this method are therefore called expeller pressed. Since the 1950s, this pressed oil has often been called "cold-pressed" oil by health food stores. This term does not accurately describe how the oil is extracted; it is actually misleading since almost all oils that are extracted through this process reach at least 130–150°F while being pressed.

The term "cold pressed" was originally used in the 1933 textbook *Food Products*, by Henry Sherman, professor of chemistry at Columbia University. Over the years health food stores have commonly used this term in order to distinguish these oils from the solvent-extracted varieties that are sold in most supermarkets. Some oils, like those derived from corn germ (corn oil) or soybeans (soybean oil), are heated to 180–240°F prior to pressing. Although heating frees the oil and makes extraction easier (also destroying the digestion-inhibiting agents in soybeans), the high temperatures reduce the nutritional content of the oil. Research done in the early 1970s has confirmed this. When heat was used to process rapeseed oil and sunflower seed oil, for example, it was discovered that they had much less vitamin E than the crude oil. Rapeseed oil contained only 65 percent as much vitamin E as its crude form, while cottonseed contained 20 percent as much as its crude form.

The Solvent-Extraction Method

This method, invented in Germany in 1870, is used to prepare most of the commercially available oil. The oil is extracted from its source by grinding its seeds and bathing them in a solvent—generally hexane, which is derived from petroleum. The resulting solvent-oil solution is boiled in order to evaporate the solvent. As undesirable as this process sounds to natural foods enthusiasts, it is the most economical method since 98 to 99 percent of the oil is extracted with very little residue remaining.

A number of other processes will take place before this
bland oil goes to the marketplace. These additional processes can be described in five steps.

1. *Degumming.* A sodium hydroxide solution is used to
    wash the oil and remove its phosphatides, including lec-
    ithin, which is considered by many to be essential to a
    healthy nervous system. Phosphatides are removed be-
    cause they may cause the oil to darken when heated.
    Most commercial oil manufacturers try to avoid any
    dark-colored oil. Apparently they feel that this color re-
    duces the commercial value of the oil.

2. *Refining.* Soap stock forms when the free fatty acids in
    the oil combine with the caustic soda. This makes the
    manufacturing of oil especially profitable for many large
    companies that manufacture soap-based cleaning prod-
    ucts as well as cooking and salad oils.

3. *Bleaching.* Bentonite (a type of clay), fuller's earth, and/
    or acid-treated clays are used to filter the oil. This
    bleaches the oil by removing the minerals and color
    components, like carotenoids and chlorophyll, and any
    remaining soap. This filtering process removes as much
    as 80 percent of the oil's iron content.

4. *Deodorization.* Hot steam coils are used to heat the oil in
    an air-free environment to 446°F. This removes more of
    the free fatty acids, aromatic oils, and other unpleasant
    odors and tastes that become evident after the first three
    steps of processing. This process leaves the oil tasteless
    and odorless, or "deodorized."

5. *Hydrogenation.* This optional step is the hardening of the
    oil into margarine or a solid cooking mixture like Crisco
    shortening. This process, accomplished by the addition
    of hydrogen to the liquid oil, is known as hydrogena-
    tion and is generally considered detrimental to health.

One of the problems with the processing of oils is that
they tend to become unstable. The quality of the oil is

greatly affected by the amount of heat, light, and oxygen that is involved during processing and packaging. Most commercial oils are refined and processed in a way that brings many of these factors into play, ultimately decreasing the nutritional value and flavor of these oils.

You can obtain the highest quality of expeller-pressed oil (also called cold-pressed oil) by extracting it in the dark in an oxygen-free environment without the use of heat (if possible). Whenever heat is necessary for processing the oil, it should be kept at an absolute minimum. All so-called cold-pressed oils may not be prepared under these strict standards. These naturally processed oils usually still contain nutritional factors such as lecithin, carotenoids (provitamin A), vitamin E, and chlorophyll as well as copper, calcium, iron, magnesium and other minerals that are not found in solvent-processed oil. How the different types of processing will affect the quality of the oil will be discussed further in Chapter 6, "Getting to Know Your Fats and Oils."

Many consumers believe that the small natural foods companies manufacture and package the expeller- or cold-pressed oils that they buy in the natural foods store, but this is not the case. Vegetable oils are often extracted by large billion-dollar companies, such as Kraft Foods, General Mills, and Hunt-Wesson Foods, and then sold to smaller packagers. Many of these packagers are the companies that market oil with the misleading "cold pressed" description on the label. A truly reputable packager will avoid using the deceiving term "cold pressed," since these oils are often a combination of expeller-pressed oil integrated with oil that has been chemically extracted, bleached, deodorized, and chemically preserved.

Once expeller-pressed oils are extracted, they are generally bottled and stored, but this is not the case with solvent-extracted oils. The use of the label "cold pressed" does not guarantee anything other than the fact that the oil was probably prepared without solvents. The pressure process generally squeezes out 95 percent of the oil. When buying oils it is best to look for the term "expeller pressed" on the label.

Differences Between Traditional and Mass-Produced Oils.

Due to the ways in which the oils are extracted and processed, there are many differences between the mass-produced oils of today and traditional oils. Some of these include:

- *Taste and aroma.* Traditional oils have a rich, full taste and aroma. Mass-produced oils have a bland taste and virtually no aroma.

- *Use of pesticides.* Traditional oils are grown naturally without sprays. Mass-produced oils have pesticide residues. These can interfere with nerve function. Some of these sprays may cause cancer and lower general vitality.

- *Use of chemical solvents.* The only ingredient of traditional oils is oil. Mass-produced oils may contain chemical solvent residues. Many of these solvents are nerve depressants and lung irritants.

- *Presence of antioxidants.* Traditional oils have naturally occurring antioxidants. When oils are mass-produced, synthetic antioxidants including BHT, BHA, citric acid, and methyl silicone are added. These are added to improve the oil's shelf life, but are foreign to your body's enzyme systems. These synthetic antioxidants may cause inefficient energy production in addition to impaired cellular respiration and metabolism. Over an extended period of time, these factors may contribute to poor general health and disease.

- *Use of heat.* Traditional oils involve minimal heat in production. Mass-produced oils are produced under very high temperatures with loss of many nutritional factors and natural antioxidants. Among those substances removed are lecithin, vitamins A and E, minerals, chlorophyll, and various aromatic and volatile compounds.

COMMERCIAL USES OF FATS AND OILS

Throughout history the availability of fats has enabled man to create light, shelter, and heat. Without fats man could not have lubricated his tools, nor could he have created many of the oils and perfumes used to beautify himself and for religious ceremonies. For no other use, however, have fats been more important to man than as a food. Fats are found in various amounts in plants and animals. Meat fats are also added to food products to enhance their flavor.

It is the fat in beef that helps give it a flavor distinctive from other types of meat. Years ago, in New York City, the price of beef rose so high that some distributors feared that people might buy horse meat for their burgers. In order to make their beef product seem more beeflike in taste, they added beef fat to the product. Needless to say, the horse meat did not sell well.

Oils may be used for flavor, aroma, and texture, or to alter a food product cosmetically. They are used on salads and in cooking, shortenings, and margarines. The many uses of different types of oils are discussed in detail in Chapter 6, "Getting to Know Your Fats and Oils."

Although excessive consumption of certain types of fat can contribute to disease, other types of fat in the proper amounts are essential for good health. You will understand the role fats and oils play in good nutrition after you learn how these nutrients work in the body in Chapter 2.

2

How Fats and Oils Work in the Body

Despite all the negative publicity surrounding fats, they are an essential part of the human diet. Of all the nutrients that we read about including vitamins and minerals, only three nutrients are a source of energy to the body: protein, carbohydrates, and fat. Of these three, fat supplies over twice the amount of calories (energy) than that provided by the other two.

Much of the negativity associated with fats has resulted from the fact that certain types of fat contribute to a number of health problems. To perceive all fats and oils in this light, however, is inaccurate. There is food fat (the fat you eat) and body fat (the fat your body produces and stores). Both food fat and body fat are essential to good health. The danger arises from certain undesirable food fats that have an adverse effect on your body chemistry. Excessive body fat can be dangerous to good health as well.

Many people do not realize that you do not produce body fat simply from eating too much fat; it is created from an excessive calorie intake. Thus, your body can convert any food, whether it's a source of fat, carbohydrates, or protein, and store it in the form of body fat. You can see that overeating in general, not merely overeating fats, can lead to excessive storage of body fat.

HOW DOES YOUR BODY STORE FAT?

Unused energy (calories) is stored in the body as fat. This stored energy may be used in two ways: for voluntary or involuntary activity. (In recent years certain functions thought to have been totally involuntary, such as certain muscle responses, were found to respond occasionally in a voluntary manner. This has especially come to light with research on biofeedback.) Voluntary activities include those physical actions that the individual can control such as walking, running, sitting, writing, bicycling, and other athletic exercises. Involuntary activities include the automatic functioning of the body's organs: the kidneys, liver, heart, stomach, lungs, and spleen, among others.

HOW ARE FATS CLASSIFIED?

It is not hard to become confused with all the different types of fats and fat-related compounds that we hear about. Although there are many ways to define specific types of fat, some terms are used more than others. You need to become familiar with these terms in order to understand what fats do in your body. A fatty acid is the component of fat that is responsible for its saturated or unsaturated quality. The fatty acids that *cannot* be produced by the body are called *essential* fatty acids. Those that *can* be produced by the body are called *nonessential* fatty acids. In addition, fats can be found in more than one form and are derived from different sources. *Saturated* fats are those that remain solid at room temperature and are generally derived from animals. *Polyunsaturated* fats, on the other hand, are liquid at room temperature and primarily come from vegetables.

For many years a classification system was used to differentiate fats. Fats were divided into three basic groups: simple lipids, compound lipids, and derived lipids. Simple lipids contain triglycerides (also called neutral fats) and waxes. Diverse combinations of triglycerides and other components form compound lipids. Fat substances called derived lipids are derived from simple and compound lipids through a process known as hydrolysis. In hydrolysis there is a type of enzymatic breakdown. Three common types of derived lipids include glycerol, fatty acids, and steroids.

Although these three categories can themselves be divided into even more subcategories, the discussion of these subcategories will be kept at a minimum for the purpose of simplicity.

Unlike the classification of fats used in the past, today we typically divide blood fats or lipids into the following three major groups: cholesterol (the most highly publicized), phospholipids, and triglycerides. Each of these blood fats will form a lipoprotein when it is combined with a protein. The resulting lipoprotein may be one of these four main types: high-density, low-density, or very-low-density lipoprotein or chylomicrons.

Because fats are made up of various lipids (fatlike substances) including triglycerides, phospholipids, sterols, fat-soluble vitamins, and tocopherols, you will soon see that fats can appear in many forms and combinations.

Triglycerides

Most of the food fats are classified as **triglycerides**. Triglycerides are a combination of glycerol and various fatty acids. All fats and oils are mixtures of varying levels of triglycerides. In terms of nutritional needs, the level of triglycerides is not as important as the type and amount of each fatty acid, since the body separates the triglycerides into fatty acids and glycerol, and then reorganizes the parts into triglycerides again according to the body's requirements. These fats are the primary way in which your body can store energy for future use. Egg yolks and edible seeds store energy in the form of triglycerides. When you are eating a healthy, well-balanced diet, the triglycerides will also serve as the storage vehicle for linoleic acid (LA) and linolenic acid (LNA), two essential fatty acids. The type of oil or fat will be determined by the structure of the fat and the manner in which the essential fatty acids are situated in that fat. The structure and positions of each component of beef fat may be different from that found in butter or fruits and vegetables. Some are saturated while others are unsaturated.

Fat serves both a metabolic and structural function in the body. Fat is used by the body metabolically to store energy. Polyunsaturated fats are essential because they contain fatty acids that are necessary to synthesize hormones, utilize vitamins A and D, and maintain the membranes surrounding each cell.

Functions of Triglycerides and Fats

The fatty acids in triglycerides serve as fuel that enables your organs (except for the brain) to perform their essential functions. The brain requires glucose, which can be manufactured from glycerol or protein, as its fuel. There are times when your body must rely on its stored energy: when you are between meals, while you are asleep, when you are exerting yourself during exercise or heavy physical labor, when you are pregnant, and when there is famine. Unlike human beings, plants do not have a stored energy system. This would become evident if your house plants were not watered or did not receive enough light. They simply would stop growing without an external energy source. The most basic nutritional function of fat is to supply the body with a highly concentrated source of energy. Neither protein nor carbohydrates can adequately compare with fat in this respect. In fact, fat provides more than twice the "fuel value" of either of these two. Fat is your body's most effective way of storing energy.

If you were to consume excessive amounts of a substance such as sugar, your body could convert it to fat so that the toxicity of the substance would be reduced. Fats in the form of triglycerides offer the body a safety mechanism, a means of converting potentially toxic substances into stored neutral substances. Although it is necessary for proper brain functioning, high levels of sugar can be toxic. By enabling the body to convert any excess sugar to triglycerides, fat protects the body and then releases the sugar again in a safe form when the body requires it.

Fat is such a good source of stored energy due to its low solubility, high concentration, and high density. When necessary, your body has the ability to convert carbohydrates and proteins into fat for storage purposes. The fat that is stored in your body as adipose tissue does not remain in its initial state. There is an ongoing continuous turnover and replacement of fat when necessary.

Fat also serves a structural function. It surrounds and protects the vital organs and nerves by holding them in place, by absorbing shock, and by supplying them with a general padding. In addition, there is a subcutaneous layer of fat that acts as an insulator by preventing rapid heat loss or temperature change in the body.

Are Triglycerides a Health Risk?

It is believed by many scientists that high triglyceride levels in the blood can lead to various health problems. Studies indicate that there is a correlation between these high levels and an increased risk of developing blood vessel and heart disease. Because there is no clear evidence that triglycerides directly cause atherosclerosis, an artery-clogging disease, nutritionists are still debating whether high triglyceride levels actually cause this damage or if their presence is the result of another factor that causes this disease. This is an important issue for determining proper treatment. If high triglyceride levels do not cause atherosclerosis, but are merely a symptom of this health problem, then any medical treatment used to lower high triglyceride levels would be unnecessary.

What happens when you eat more carbohydrates and sugar than your body can handle? Think about what happens when your town produces so much garbage that your local dump can't handle it. Someone or something has to handle the overflow. When your body can't use the amount of carbohydrates and sugar that has been consumed, it responds by converting the excess amounts into fat and storing them in your body. The amount of fat produced as a result, however, is often excessive and difficult for your body to store. The overload of fat is then "dumped" into the various organs and tissues of your body including the liver, kidneys, heart, arteries, and even muscles. These fatty deposits generally indicate that a fatty degeneration is taking place, since fat is generally not found in these places.

Disorders associated with fatty degeneration include diabetes, rheumatic diseases, atherosclerosis, obesity, various types of tumors, and kidney and liver degeneration. High triglyceride levels in the blood increase the probability that blood cells will adhere to each other, thus reducing the amount of oxygen that the blood can carry. The less oxygen carried by the blood, the greater the risk of cancer and other degenerative diseases.

Research has not yet been conducted to determine how the requirements for the essential fatty acids vary among individuals. It is not an exaggeration to say that the needs of a specific essential nutrient may vary tenfold or more from person to person. Factors such as stress or disease can change these requirements even more. "As with most essential nutrients, it appears likely that the optimum requirements for the essential fatty acids is higher than the minimum requirement. Five to ten percent of daily calories as LA [linoleic acid], 2% as LNA [linolenic acid] and a combined total of essential fatty acids of at least one third of the total fat consumed has been suggested as optimum."

Triglycerides are transported in the blood by lipoproteins called chylomicrons and very-low-density lipoproteins (or VLDLs). Tissue enzymes will remove the triglycerides from the VLDLs, breaking the VLDLs down into smaller particles called low-density lipoproteins (or LDLs). The role that LDLs and VLDLs play in heart disease is discussed in Chapter 5.

What Causes High Triglyceride Levels?

There are a number of reasons why triglyceride levels might be high. Among the major ones are:

- *Excessive weight.* The greater your weight is, the higher your triglyceride levels will be. If you are overweight and have high triglyceride levels, you can lower them simply by losing weight.

- *Carbohydrate sensitivity.* Consuming refined starches, sugars, and large amounts of alcohol will generally cause an increase in blood triglyceride levels.

- *Birth control pills.* Women who take oral contraceptives tend to have higher blood triglyceride levels.

- *Genetic factors.* It has been found that a genetic predisposition to elevated triglyceride levels will exist in at least one out of every twenty people.

- *Age.* It is not yet clear whether high triglyceride levels are the result of a cultural or biological factor, but it is clear that triglyceride levels rise with age. Thus, up to age thirty, your triglyceride level is considered normal if you have less than 140 milligrams of triglycerides per deciliter of blood serum.

In addition to fat, there are a number of important fat-related compounds. Among these are phospholipids and sterols (of which cholesterol is one).

Phospholipids

Whereas triglycerides are the first major group of lipids found in foods and in your body, phospholipids are the second major group. **Phospholipids**, which are a chemical combination of fatty acids, phosphorus, and nitrogen, play a major role in the structure of the organism. Although they are similar to triglycerides in many ways, phospholipids are unlike other fats and fat-related compounds in that they are water-soluble and tend to disperse over surfaces. This quality of spreading in a thin layer whenever oil and water come together enables the phospholipids to form the double-layered membrane that is the skin of every living cell.

Functions of Phospholipids

Phospholipids serve many functions. Because they form the skinlike layers of the organelles (a specialized part of a cell that functions as an organ), phospholipids act as a barrier by separating the cells from the outside world. This barrier protects the cell from foreign organisms. Together with protein, phospholipids regulate which substances can enter and leave the cell. Without phospholipids to hold the protein of the membrane in place, it wouldn't be able to perform its important functions. Certain substances can readily cross the barrier despite its efficient regulation. These include barbiturates and other prescription drugs, alcohol, and certain carcinogens.

In addition to its regulatory function, phospholipids help cholesterol and fats to dissolve in the blood, and prevent them from forming on arterial walls. They help prevent hypertension, heart and kidney failure, stroke, heart attack, and other cardiovascular disorders that can occur due to the accumulation of cholesterol and triglycerides along the walls of the arteries. Phospholipids prevent lipids from forming bubbles and rising in the blood in much the same way that cream rises to the top of milk.

Lecithin

Probably the most familiar type of phospholipid is lecithin. Lecithin was first isolated and extracted from egg yolks, and its name is derived from the Greek word for this food. Eggs are not the only source of lecithin, however. Most seed oils contain lecithin, and soybean oil is its most abundant source. It is comprised of as much as 2 percent lecithin. Whereas the lecithin in soybean oil is particularly rich in both essential fatty acids, the lecithin found in most other oils contains linoleic acid, but is lacking in linolenic acid.

Functions of Lecithin

Although the functions of lecithin are similar to those of all phospholipids, it does have others specific to it. As much as half of its fatty acid content is made up of those essential fatty acids that cannot be manufactured from other fats in the body. Lecithin prevents an accumulation of fat in the body. It acts as a detergent by emulsifying fats, breaking them up into smaller particles that are held in suspension. By emulsifying fatty substances, lecithin prevents the formation of kidney stones and gallstones and dissolves any existing stones. As an essential component of bile, lecithin also emulsifies food fats, increasing their surface area and facilitating fat digestion through enzymatic action.

In addition to its presence in bile, lecithin also assists the liver in detoxification. Improper detoxification may be a forerunner of cancer. Because of its influence on the thymus, lecithin also helps promote resistance to disease. As a phosphatide, it is involved in the prevention of cardiovascular problems and atherosclerosis as well.

Phospholipids may often have other chemical structures associated with them. Some have mysterious functions, while others have important nutritional qualities. The most commonly known of these associated factors are choline, inositol, serine, and ethanolamine. Phosphatidal choline and inositol are often found in the lecithin supplements that are available in health food stores and in other nutritional supplement formulas.

Cholesterol

Cholesterol, chemically speaking, is a waxy alcohol closely related to adrenal hormones and sex hormones. Unlike fat, which can be found in fruits, vegetables, nuts, seeds, and other vegetation, cholesterol is found only in animal foods such as eggs, poultry, meat, fish, and shellfish.

The average human body contains approximately 150,000 milligrams (150 grams) of cholesterol, most of which is located in the membranes. About 700 milligrams of cholesterol are carried in the blood. In the United States approximately 800 milligrams of cholesterol are consumed by the average person daily. Of course, these figures may vary depending on one's health, body size, and dietary patterns.

About half of the cholesterol that we obtain from food is neither absorbed nor utilized by the body. The remaining 50 percent will either be used for essential functions or may contribute to various health problems (discussed in Chapter 5). Because your body has the ability to manufacture all the cholesterol that it requires, it is not necessary to obtain cholesterol from your diet. Cells manufacture cholesterol based upon the amount required to perform vital functions. For example, when you drink alcohol, the alcohol dissolves in the membranes, giving them increased fluidity. Responding to this increased fluidity, the cell walls produce more cholesterol to reduce the membrane fluidity. As the amount of alcohol in your system diminishes, the membranes begin to harden again and cholesterol production in the cell ceases.

Cholesterol is produced not only by your cells, but also by the sex and adrenal glands, the small intestines, and the liver. The cholesterol manufactured by these organs is used for other essential functions.

Your body manufactures cholesterol from the simple fragments produced from the breakdown of proteins, sugars, and fats. If your diet is high in fat (especially saturated or other nonessential fatty acids), your body will respond by converting excess fat to cholesterol. Individuals on a diet high in fat or sugar, therefore, tend to have higher cholesterol levels than those whose diet contains less of these compounds. Whether or not this cholesterol will be detrimental to your health is largely dependent upon how it is carried in the blood.

Low-density lipoproteins (LDLs), very-low-density lipoproteins (VLDLs), and high-density lipoproteins (HDLs) play an important role in how cholesterol works in your body. Cholesterol can be carried in the blood by any of these three types of lipoprotein; however, it is now known that LDLs and VLDLs can contribute to the formation of cholesterol-thick plaques in your arteries, which may lead to cardiovascular disease. See Chapter 5, "Understanding and Reducing the Dangers of Fats and Oils," for health problems associated with LDLs and VLDLs, and for suggestions on how to reduce LDL and VLDL levels.

Functions of Cholesterol

Despite the negative publicity often received by cholesterol, there are many bodily functions that could not take place without it. The cell membranes are regulated, in part, by the amount of cholesterol present. If the cholesterol level in the cell membrane is too low, the membrane may become too fluid and begin to break down. The amount of cholesterol produced by your body compensates for changes in membrane fluidity. Membrane fluidity fluctuates according to the level of fatty acids in your body from day to day.

There are many essential vitamins, hormones, and chemical compounds that are derived from cholesterol or that require cholesterol for their manufacture. Three hormones that are manufactured from cholesterol are steroid (or sex) hormones, aldosterone, and cortisone.

Of the steroid hormones produced from cholesterol, the best known are estrogen and progesterone in women and testosterone in men. During pregnancy the placenta will manufacture cholesterol. The cholesterol is needed to produce progesterone, which keeps the pregnancy from terminating. Estrogen, progesterone, and testosterone are essential to the development and maintenance of the physical attributes associated with each sex.

Aldosterone, an adrenal corticosteroid hormone manufactured from cholesterol, maintains the balance of water in the kidneys by increasing the ability of the renal tubes to retain sodium.

Another adrenal corticosteroid hormone produced from cholesterol, called cortisone, aids in the production of glucose. This vital hormone enables your body to respond to stress by producing glucose. In stressful situations, your body will energize itself through glucose production in a response known as "fight or flight." Cortisone also helps the immune system by preventing and reducing inflammation.

Cholesterol is also used to make vitamin D, which is necessary for your body to utilize calcium and phosphorus. In addition to vitamin D, cholesterol helps to form bile acids, which ease digestion by emulsifying food fats. Interestingly, even though bile acids are derived from cholesterol, they also play an important role in discarding excess cholesterol from the body that it does not need.

FATTY ACIDS

As mentioned earlier, all fats are composed of a combination of different triglycerides. In nutrition the most important basic structural units are the fatty acids. In order to meet its own needs, your body may reorganize its glycerol and fatty acids into triglycerides when necessary.

Polyunsaturated fats are made up of various fatty acids. When your body requires fatty acids, your liver can convert certain saturated fats into polyunsaturates.

Essential Fatty Acids

Fatty acids are generally categorized as essential or nonessential. Historically, only those nutrients whose absence was shown to result in a particular disorder were deemed important. For example, it was discovered in 1930 that if an animal's diet were devoid of fat, certain symptoms would arise: poor reproduction, low resistance to infection, scaly skin, slow growth, and certain chemical changes in the blood. Biochemists soon found that these symptoms could have been prevented and could even be corrected by adding certain fatty acids to the diet—the **essential fatty acids**. Essential fatty acids used to be known as "vitamin F." As in animals, there are certain fatty acids that your body cannot synthesize or manufacture from other fats which are essential to good health. These are called essential fatty acids (EFAs).

A fatty acid is considered essential given *one* of these two reasons:

1. The body is unable to manufacture it and must obtain it through the diet.

2. A deficiency or absence of the fatty acid results in a specific disease. (For example, a deficiency of linoleic acid in infants can cause a certain type of eczema.)

There are three essential fatty acids that fit this definition—linoleic acid, linolenic acid, and arachidonic acid. Without these fatty acids, certain essential body functions cannot take place. Of these three, linoleic acid is the most important because it is the only one that strictly fits the specific definitions of an essential fatty acid. Linolenic acid (in the presence of vitamin B_6) and arachidonic acid can be manufactured from linoleic acid. Arachidonic acid is particularly important to reactions involving fat-protein metabolism in the cell nucleus. Since this fatty acid does not have a vegetable source, those vegetarians who are unable to convert linoleic acid must take supplementary amounts of linolenic and arachidonic acids. Linolenic acid is generally considered less essential because it has a small but limited effect in eliminating some of the symptoms traditionally associated with an essential fatty acid deficiency. Because linolenic and arachidonic acids can be converted from linoleic acid, they do not necessarily have to be obtained from food.

The Function of Essential Fatty Acids

There are a number of body functions that require essential fatty acids (EFAs). All body membranes require EFAs for their construction. Without them, cholesterol and protein would be unable to repair old cell membranes or to construct new cell membranes. EFAs also make up lipoprotein and phospholipid complexes.

Essential fatty acids help to strengthen the basic structure of cells and capillaries. By promoting fibrinolytic activity and prolonging blood-clotting time, EFAs allow cuts and wounds to heal. These vital nutrients also assist in the manufacture of hemoglobin. By combining with cholesterol, EFAs also form cholesterol esters. The essential fatty acids help to remove excess cholesterol from the body, lowering serum cholesterol levels.

Although it is not clearly understand exactly how the body utilizes essential fatty acids, it is known that they are responsible for transporting oxygen from the lungs to the exact location in the body where it is needed. Because of their chemical structure, EFAs attract oxygen. Consequently, they play an essential role in keeping oxygen in the cell membranes. EFAs also prevent bacteria and viruses from growing, since these organisms cannot grow well in the presence of oxygen.

Because of their role in tissue oxygenation, EFAs also greatly reduce the amount of time needed for fatigued muscles to recover after exercise. Besides allowing tissues access to oxygen, they also make calcium available for use by the tissues and elevate calcium levels in the bloodstream.

In addition to their many other functions, essential fatty acids are involved in all glandular secretions in the body including the production of adrenal hormones. They help promote healthy hair and skin. By increasing the body's metabolic rate, EFAs accelerate the rate at which the body burns calories and reduces body fat. As a source of energy, they also help to maintain body temperature. They are required for the generation of electrical currents necessary to maintain a regular heartbeat as well.

Prostaglandin Production

EFAs have an essential role as preliminary agents to the production of a group of hormonelike substances called **prostaglandins**. These compounds not only regulate many essential tissue functions, they also control every organ in the body. Although they differ from hormones in that they are not secreted by the glands, prostaglandins do act as regulators and messengers. Because prostaglandins are not stored in the body, EFAs are essential to their production. Each cell keeps tiny amounts of EFAs and produces prostaglandins from them as they are needed.

The name prostaglandins came about because these compounds were originally found in high concentrations in the prostate gland. It is now known that there are at least thirty-six different prostaglandins with a wide range of functions, and that much of their activity can be attributed to the EFAs. Apparently, this is a result of the conversion of EFAs to prostaglandins. Recent research has indicated that prostaglandins are vital to the body's immune system.

EFAs cannot efficiently produce prostaglandins without the presence of certain specific enzymes to act as catalysts. These enzymes, in turn, cannot act without the presence of certain vitamins and minerals, especially the antioxidants (vitamin E and selenium), lecithin, vitamin B_6, and vitamin A. All of these nutrients support the function of the EFAs in the body by reducing oxidation.

Deficiency Symptoms

Whereas deficiencies of essential fatty acids were generally thought to be rare, many experts now believe that the condition may be more widespread. Many of the individuals exhibiting particular symptoms also had abnormally low levels of essential fatty acids in the blood and/or in the tissues.

Because of its involvement in numerous body functions, there are many health problems associated with a deficiency of linoleic acid. Those with low levels of this essential nutrient commonly suffer from the following symptoms: acne, arthritis, behavioral changes, circulatory and heart problems, gallbladder problems, retarded growth, poor healing of wounds, kidney degeneration, miscarriage in females, muscle tremors, prostatitis, skin eruptions appearing as eczema, sterility in males, and thirstiness from abnormal water loss through the skin.

A deficiency of linolenic acid can also result in several problems including poor growth, impaired learning ability, tingling in the legs and arms, poor motor coordination, and impaired vision. All of these symptoms will clear up when adequate amounts of this essential fatty acid is returned to the diet. Long-term deficiencies of essential fatty acids can result in death.

Research on the essential fatty acids has not been easy, especially since they are easily destroyed. (Linolenic acid is more sensitive than linoleic acid.) Of the forty-five known essential nutrients, your body requires and contains more linoleic acid than any other. Although researchers are not exactly certain how much linoleic acid the body requires, it seems as if three to six grams a day or 1 to 2 percent of your daily caloric intake will prevent deficiency symptoms. A larger intake of this essential fatty acid, however, is recommended for optimum health.

Essential fatty acids can be obtained from a variety of seeds and plants. The best sources of EFAs include flaxseed oil, safflower oil, and evening primrose oil. Unfortunately, both safflower and evening primrose oil contain only linoleic acid; they do not have any linolenic acid.

The minimum requirements for EFAs, as for all essential nutrients, will vary from person to person due to many factors including stress, hormonal differences between men and women, physical activity, and diet. Diet, in particular, can affect your requirements for essential fatty acids. The more obese a person is and the greater his intake of olive oil and saturated fatty acids, the higher his EFA requirements will be. Also, without a well-balanced diet, your body may not be able to use the essential fatty acids properly. For example, certain other nutrients are necessary for linoleic acid to function properly in your body. These nutrients include vitamins B_3, B_6, and C, zinc, and to a lesser degree vitamin A.

HOW ARE FATS DIGESTED?

Fats are digested in two different ways: mechanically and chemically. Mechanical digestion begins when you chew your food. The food is broken up into very small particles and moistened so that it can pass easily into the stomach. In the stomach the food is crushed further through a muscular action called **peristalsis**.

Peristalsis mechanically mixes the fats with other stomach contents. Unlike proteins, there is no specific enzyme in the stomach to digest fat. As gastric enzymes work on the other stomach nutrients, they are separated from the fat, making it ready for the small intestine. It is in the small intestine where the chemical digestion of the fat begins.

Once the fat enters the small intestine, chemical agents from the small intestine, the pancreas, and the liver and gallbladder work to digest the fat. When fat enters the duodenum, the beginning portion of the small intestine, it stimulates the glands in the walls of the intestine. This causes the secretion of cholecystokinin, a hormone that in turn stimulates the contraction of the gallbladder, the relaxation of the sphincter, and the secretion through the common bile duct of bile salts into the intestine.

The Role of Bile in Digestion

Bile, which is produced in the liver and stored in the gallbladder, is important for the digestion of fats. Emulsification is important if the fats are to be prepared for enzymatic digestion; bile is an emulsifier of fats. Two of the most important benefits of emulsification are:

1. Emulsification breaks the fat into fine particles (globules) that bring the surface area of the fat into greater contact with fat-digesting enzymes.

2. Emulsification also reduces the surface tension of fat globules, thus making enzyme penetration easier. This process can be likened to the wetting action of detergents when you are washing your clothes.

In addition to these two factors, the bile salts also create an alkaline medium that is important for the fat-digesting enzyme, lipase, to function effectively.

The Role of Pancreatic Enzymes in Digestion

Pancreatic juice contains the powerful enzyme, steapsin, which is a type of lipase. Step by step, steapsin removes one fatty acid at a time from the glycerol base of neutral fats. Each of these steps is slow and succeedingly difficult. The end products of fat digestion are (in the order of separation) fatty acids, diglycerides, monoglycerides, and glycerol.

For a summary of fat digestion in successive parts of the gastrointestinal tract, see Table 2.1. This table describes the movement of fat through the digestive system. The digestive organs, their role in digestion, and the specific enzymes associated with each organ are listed.

When your intake of fat exceeds your body's requirements, obesity and other health problems result. Eating the right amount of fats is important for good health. Dietary fat must be regulated to avoid excess weight gain. Because obesity is one of the greatest health risks facing Americans today, the next chapter has been devoted to helping you achieve and maintain a healthy weight through the creation of an individualized dietary program.

Table 2.1   Fat Digestion

Place of Action	Enzymes for Fat Digestion	Enzyme Source	Action
Mouth	None	NA	Mechanical breakdown of food; mastication.
Stomach	None	NA	Mechanical separation of fats.
Small intestine	Bile	Gallbladder	Emulsifies fats.
	Lipase (steapsin)	Pancreas	Converts triglycerides first to di- and monoglycerides, then to fatty acids and glycerol.
	Cholesterol esterase	Pancreas	Converts free cholesterol and fatty acids to cholesterol esters.
	Lecithinase	Intestine	Converts lecithin to fatty acids, glycerol, phosphoric acid, and choline.

3
Dietary Fat and Obesity

The average American obtains about 17 percent of his total caloric intake from saturated fats, and has a total cholesterol intake of about 500 milligrams each day. Although the general recommendations for fat intake may change from year to year, many nutritionists recommend that your fat intake be no more than 30 percent of your daily caloric intake, of which no more than 10 percent should be of the saturated type. Compared to carbohydrates and proteins, fats are the most concentrated source of calories, regardless of whether they are derived from an animal or vegetable source. (Fats contain twice the amount of calories as carbohydrates or proteins, gram for gram.)

Before you can begin to regulate the amounts and types of fat in your diet, you should understand the differences between saturated, unsaturated, and polyunsaturated fats.

WHAT IS THE DIFFERENCE BETWEEN SATURATED AND UNSATURATED FAT?

Fats are often described either as saturated or polyunsaturated. Anyone who reads the newspaper or watches television is often presented with commercials extolling the high polyunsaturate content of this or that product. Saturated fats are hard at room temperature and are prevalent in red meat, butter, cheese, sour cream, and coconut oil. Even certain margarines that claim to contain no cholesterol may be artifically saturated. Haven't you ever seen margarine labels listing hardened, partially hardened, or hydrogenated oil as the main ingredient?

Unlike saturated fats, polyunsaturated fats (which are commonly called oils) take on a liquid state at room temperature. The most popular of the polyunsaturated fats include olive, peanut, canola, safflower, and sunflower oils.

As you already know, all fats have a certain amount of carbon, hydrogen, and oxygen molecules in them. The carbon atoms of fatty acids form what might be called a chain. Different chains of carbon will carry different amounts of hydrogen. When all of the carbon atoms are filled with the available hydrogen atoms and unable to hold any more, these carbon atoms are said to be *saturated* with hydrogen atoms. It is from this concept that the name **saturated fats** is derived.

Although many fats are saturated, all saturated fatty acids are not the same. Since some carbon chains are longer than others, the level of saturation will vary. It is known, for example, that the length of the carbon chain correlates to its melting point and hardness. The longer the carbon chain is in a saturated fatty acid (SFA), the higher its melting point will be and the harder it will be as well. About 10 percent of the total fatty acid content of butter and milk fat is comprised of short-chain saturated fatty acids. Some of these short-chain SFAs are also found in coconut oil. If a fatty acid has less than ten carbons on its chain, then the fatty acid will be liquid at body temperature. Most oils and fats are fat-soluble because they dissolve in other oils and fats, but not in water. Short-chain fatty acids such as butyric acid that do dissolve in water are called water-soluble.

To determine whether a molecule is water-soluble, you may simply note the length of the carbon chain. The longer the length of its carbon chain, the less apt the molecule is to be water-soluble. Most of the fatty acids found in butter and milk fat are of the long-chain variety. It is known that these long-chain fatty acids may contribute to certain health problems.

Saturated fatty acids have certain characteristics in common that ultimately may contribute to cardiovascular disease and other diseases involving fatty degeneration. In addition to being insoluble in water, saturated fatty acids tend to stick together and, if hard, to form plaques. Long-chain SFAs are useful to the body in that they build cell membranes and prevent potentially harmful unsaturated fatty acids in the membranes from negatively interacting with each other. When the dietary intake of long-chain saturated fatty acids is high, however, the plaques that they tend to form will often stick together and deposit in the cells, organs, and arteries. A plaque may be formed from protein and cholesterol and deposited along your arteries. Thus, the higher your intake of long-chain SFAs, the greater your health risk.

Both monounsaturated fatty acids (as found in olive oil) and saturated fatty acids have been found to decrease the supply of oxygen essential to the tissues (anoxia). Thus, too high an intake of either of these fatty acids may contribute to various forms of fatty degeneration.

Although saturated fat is often associated with red meat, it is found in various foods—both animal and vegetable (palm kernel and coconut). What types of saturated fats are found in the foods we eat?

Red meats, such as beef and mutton, generally have more long-chain saturated fat than other animal fats. Although pork has more total fat than beef, a lower percentage of its total fat content is made up of long-chain SFAs. In comparison to red meat, poultry has a much lower total fat content. Most of the fat that poultry does contain is unsaturated. If you eat the skin, however, the total fat content will be as high as that contained in beef flank steak or pork loin. In addition, a higher percentage of the total fat content of dairy products (those containing whole milk) consists of long-chain SFAs.

The amount of saturated fats in your diet should generally be kept at a minimal level since they have been implicated as a contributing factor to a number of medical problems; however, there is one saturated fat that may be an exception.

Recent preliminary studies conducted by Dr. Andrea Bonanome and Dr. Scott M. Grundy at the University of Texas Southwestern Medical Center in Dallas indicate that stearic acid, one of the most prevalent types of saturated fat found in chocolate and beef, may not only lower cholesterol levels in the blood, but also lessen the effect of the cholesterol produced by other saturated fats in these same foods. This study was conducted in a laboratory setting using artificial liquid diets, and so does not necessarily reflect what would happen in a normal dietary situation. The results of this study have not yet been announced, so don't abandon your low-fat diet for a steak burger topped with sour cream dressing!

Very often you will hear someone say, "I no longer eat red meat," in order to indicate that they have eliminated beef, veal, pork, and lamb from their diet. The term "red meat" refers to the original color of beef before it has been cooked, even though it becomes brown as it is cooked.

Many factors determine whether a particular type of meat has a high fat content. These include how long the meat has been cooked and how much fat has been trimmed from it before cooking. Facts about the animal itself such as how much it had exercised, which part of the animal the meat is from, and how it had been fed are also relevant. Certain parts of the animal contain more fat than others. Those beef cattle that have been raised in grain feedlots also have a higher fat content than the range-fed cattle.

The flesh of fish is generally lower in fat than the flesh of other foods (even skinless chicken), and most of it is unsaturated. The fish and shellfish with the lowest fat and cholesterol content are clams, cod, flounder, haddock, monkfish, ocean perch, scallops, most shark excluding spiney dogfish, and swordfish.

The information about red meat and the fat content of beef, veal, pork, lamb, and fish will be relevant when you are regulating the amount of fat in your diet.

REDUCING FAT INTAKE, SATURATED FATTY ACIDS, AND CHOLESTEROL

Even if you don't have a weight problem, it's unwise to consume large amounts of calories in the form of fat. High-fat diets have been implicated as a possible cause of heart disease and cancer of the colon and breast. (This will be discussed in further detail in Chapter 5.)

Skimming the fat from your diet can be relatively painless. You can begin with a few simple gestures. Reduce the amount of butter on your bread, mayonnaise on your sandwich, and dressing on your salad.

Stop deep-frying your food and eliminate bacon, ham, and sausage from your breakfast menu. After you have removed the "visible fat" that accounts for 40 to 50 percent of all the fats you eat, you can start working on the hidden fats. You know which ones I mean—the flakey pie crust, the cheese sauces that go on your vegetables, and the nachos you get at the mall.

Imagine what is included in a typical diet—eggs and coffee for breakfast and white bread, burgers, and French fries for afternoon or evening meals. Now imagine that the person on this typical diet has decided to reduce his fat intake without eliminating too much from his diet. He is not necessarily interested in natural foods, but recognizes the risk of a diet that is too high in fat.

OBESITY

Obesity may be the greatest health risk that we face today. Among the hazards associated with obesity is a greater potential for many health problems, including back problems that result from weak abdominal muscles which put unnecessary stress on the back muscles to maintain the back in an upright position, gallbladder disease, arthritis, diabetes, heart disease, hypertension, and a weakening of the immune system that increases the risk of infection.

The majority of weight problems are the result of poor nutritional habits. It is also true that big bones, thyroid and other metabolic difficulties, psychological factors, and even genetic factors may account for obesity in some cases; however, these are relatively uncommon.

Although it seems as if Americans are obsessed with losing weight, their general exercise and dietary habits do not reflect these intentions. The level of weight-loss obsession in this country is clearly demonstrated by the fact that there are over 28,000 diets on the public record and that 65 percent of the population in the United States starts a new diet at least once each year.

How Do You Know if You Are Overweight?

A person is considered overweight if he weighs 10 to 20 percent above his ideal body weight. Obesity is now recognized by many nutritionists and physicians as the nation's number one health problem. Some estimates indicate that 25 to 45 percent of adults over thirty are overweight.

How can you avoid becoming overweight? In order to maintain your weight, your intake of calories must equal your energy output. If you want to lose weight, your caloric intake must be less than the amount of energy that you expend. If your goal is to gain weight, your caloric intake must exceed your energy output. Any unused calories will be stored in your body as fat.

Where your body tends to store fat can be of significance. If much of your body fat is located in your abdomen, you are at greater risk for diabetes, high blood pressure, and heart attacks. Your goal, then, is to try to maintain a safe weight through a healthy diet and plenty of exercise. As you get older, of course, your dietary and exercise requirements will change as your metabolism slows.

Due to some essential differences between men and women, caloric intake and hormonal changes will affect the way in which they gain weight. As a woman becomes older, she will require fewer calories to maintain her weight. After a woman has experienced menopause, her energy requirements will be about 15 percent less than when she was in her twenties; yet, with the exception of iron, her requirements for most nutrients will remain the same. Because of these changes, older women can afford fewer "empty calories" than men. Your caloric requirements will depend upon your gender, physical size, and activity level. For example, a six-foot man can eat and absorb several hundred more calories without gaining weight than a five-foot-five-inch woman. Researchers at the University of Michigan have discovered a correlation between the age at which a woman matures and her weight. They found that women who began menstruating at age eleven or younger were 30 percent fatter when they reached the age of thirty than those who began menstruating at a later age.

As you age, the manner in which your body holds fat will change. For example, it is possible that even though some people have maintained the same weight for twenty years, their weight may now be redistributed around the midsection: they are now considered to be overweight even though they weren't twenty years ago at the same weight. You may even be overweight while standard height-weight charts tell you that you're within a healthy or normal range. If more than 25 percent of your body weight is fat, then you are obese.

Although there are certain nutritional and dietary factors that might affect weight gain, such as allergic reaction, food sensitivity, or supplementation with certain amino acids, the use of special foods or special food supplements will not generally reduce weight.

In recent years I have read some articles that have referred to fat as beautiful and some that have proclaimed that thin is good and fat is bad. Whether you should be fat or thin is more than an issue of aesthetics. When you carry excess fat on your body, you are statistically more prone to certain dangers. Many experts believe that if you hold more fat in your abdomen than in other areas of your body, you have a greater potential for obesity.

HOW TO LOSE WEIGHT INTELLIGENTLY AND EFFECTIVELY

Just about any diet will help you lose weight. It is important to remember that losing weight is not your only goal. You want to lose weight in a healthy, well-balanced manner, and then keep it off.

Losing weight takes strong determination, a strong support network, and a lot of hard work. As your weight drops during a diet, so does your body's caloric requirements. Thus, the greater your weight loss, the lower your daily caloric intake will have to be in order for you to continue to lose weight at the same pace. You must, therefore, be motivated over a period of time in order to successfully lose weight. For example, a moderately active female weighing 135 pounds can lose about a pound each week on a 1,500-calorie diet. Once she has slimmed to 125 pounds, however, she must consume no more than 1,200 calories a day to maintain this rate of loss.

These changes in caloric requirements are a result of changes that take place in the dieter's metabolic rate. Because of these changes, a long-term low-calorie diet may have limited effectiveness for some individuals. Recent research has indicated that despite very strict low-calorie diets, there are certain obese individuals who are unable to lose weight after their initial weight loss. They can no longer lose weight because their metabolic rates have dropped to "protect" them from starving. An article appearing in *The New York Times* in March 1987 states:

> New studies indicate that for many obese people, relatively small weight losses—often only 10 percent of body weight—can correct a tendency to-

ward diabetes or high blood pressure. Thus major health risks associated with obesity might be countered with modest losses of 10 to 25 pounds that are easier to maintain.

Beware of Unbalanced Weight-Loss Practices

One of the limitations of "crash diets" and nutritionally unbalanced weight-loss practices is their long-term ineffectiveness. All too often, the dieter gains back all of the weight he has lost from "liquid diets," excessively rigid menus, and other extreme approaches. There are certain approaches that you should avoid and some facts that you should be aware of while developing a healthy weight-control program.

Any of the following could be a giveaway that the diet will be unsafe or ineffective (and should be avoided!):

• Beware of rigid menus. Few people will ever stick to a program like this for any length of time.

• Beware of certain foods that will magically make fat disappear without any caloric control.

• Beware of diets that promise a large amount of weight loss quickly. The initial weight lost at the beginning of almost all diets that restrict calories, carbohydrates, and salt is simply water weight. In fact, studies have shown that the faster you lose weight, the more likely it is that you will regain it.

• Beware of excessively high- or low-protein diets. When your protein intake is too high, you increase your risk for many serious illnesses including cancer and heart disease. Liquid high-protein diets tend to be too high in protein and too low in calories. Some side effects experienced on such a diet might include constipation, cramps, bad breath, and hair loss. On the other hand, when your diet is deficient in protein for too long a period, the body may begin digesting its own organs and muscles.

• Beware of any diet that makes you feel very weak or results in either cracked nails or excessive loss of hair. If this happens, there is a good chance that certain aspects of your diet are very unhealthy.

- Beware of diets of less than 1,000-1,200 calories a day. When you cut back your caloric intake too rapidly as you do on many diets or when you fast, you may cause your body to reduce the number of calories it burns. When this happens, you may find that you are still not losing weight, despite your low-calorie diet. The more compulsive and extreme a diet tends to be, the less likely it is that it will help you take weight off and keep it off.

- Beware of fasting to lose weight. Many people see fasting as the best way to lose weight. Although fasting can be a very powerful, natural healing tool, it is not a wise choice for a productive weight-control program. Fasting will neither help you learn how to make proper food choices nor how to eat moderately—the two most important dietary factors for effective weight loss. Fasting can also lead to serious difficulties. Long fasts that are not properly supervised can cause kidney failure, blood pH problems, liver malfunction, and electrolyte depletion, and they can reduce the intestinal absorption of nutrients and the digestive enzyme level in the stomach and intestines. In addition, the most effective, permanent weight-loss program is one that will teach you to eat in moderation and plan well-balanced meals. Just as overeating involves compulsive behavior, fasting is a compulsive way to lose weight and should, therefore, be avoided by dieters.

Nutritional Considerations

Many orthodox nutritionists and researchers have argued for years that all calories are equal and that one food is not any better at promoting weight loss than another food of the same caloric value. Recent research, however, now indicates that if you obtain you calories from fat, you are less likely to lose weight than you would be with an equal amount of calories from starch. According to an article from *The New York Times*:

> Dr. Elliot Danforth of the University of Vermont in Burlington explained that dietary fat is the only nutrient that can beat a direct path to the body's fat deposits. Only 2.5 percent of the calories in fat are needed to accomplish this. Starches, on the other hand, "cost" about 25 percent of ingested calories to be stored as fat, and only about 1 percent of ingested carbohydrates end up as body fat. . . . Simply switching from a high-fat diet to one high in carbohydrates, without actually lowering total caloric intake, can result in a net caloric loss to the body.

Changing Your Dietary Patterns

Although will power more often than not seems to determine whether a weight-loss program is effective, there are many things you can do to increase your chances for success. You can choose the approach that is best for you for a healthy weight-control program.

There are a number of strategies that you can use in order to successfully combat too much body fat. One way to lose weight effectively is to choose a vegetarian diet. This type of diet generally has a lower intake of fat. Because this diet is also high in fiber and uses lots of low-calorie vegetables, you will generally become full before you have had a chance to consume many calories.

Drinking as much as eight glasses of fluid (water, broth, or cleansing herb teas) each day can also help you lose weight. These fluids will reduce your hunger pangs and cleanse your body of toxic substances that gather as you burn body fat.

You should try to avoid foods that are high in calories. These include ones that are high in fat and heavily processed foods containing hydrogenated and partially hydrogenated fats. Some foods that are generally considered healthy, such as hard cheeses, nuts, avocados, and coconuts, should be avoided due to the large percentage of calories that they obtain from fat. Eat moderate amounts of protein and little or no saturated fat. Instead, try foods like fresh fruits and vegetables, whole grains, and beans. These are high in fiber and contain complex carbohydrates. As much as 30 percent of the calories found in foods high in complex carbohydrates are not absorbed and will pass through your body without adding to your caloric intake. This approach is especially effective because you tend to feel more satisfied after meals with a smaller caloric intake. Weight loss will be slow and steady.

The way in which you prepare foods will also affect weight gain. Broil, steam, or bake all foods that are not eaten raw. Do not add extra oil or butter. Prepare small portions of food; you will be more tempted to finish a larger portion if it is in front of you. You should also avoid keeping snack foods in your house that are not part of your weight-loss program. Some people keep them around for friends who may "drop by." This will not work for you. If you don't have any of these snacks, you won't be tempted to eat them. Your friends will just have to obtain their potato chips elsewhere. Instead of keeping these undesirable snack foods in the house, you can bake several potatoes ahead of time and keep them in the refrigerator. When you are hungry for a snack, you can cut one in half and have it with a tablespoon of yogurt.

It's a good idea to keep a diary of what you eat, so that you can confirm your daily caloric intake. You may be surprised to find that the seemingly small amounts of food you have eaten actually contain more fat or calories than you have dreamed! Set up a meal plan every morning so that you will not eat spontaneously. If your lunch is scheduled for one o'clock, eat it then and not earlier. This type of meal scheduling will help you keep your commitments concerning food. You should also try to avoid activities, such as reading or watching television, while you are eating. If you eat while you are seated comfortably so that you may concentrate on your food instead of while you are standing and involved in some other activity, then you will have a greater awareness of your food and your relationship to it.

You can increase your motivation to lose weight by keeping reminders of when you were thinner, such as photos and smaller-sized clothing, within view. Exercise on a regular basis and do not reward yourself with food.

Try to divide your caloric intake into as many as six very small meals a day. By eating many small meals, you are more likely to avoid sweets and sugary snacks between meals. In addition, the production of insulin and resulting body fat that takes place with large meals will be reduced. Eating slowly is also beneficial. If you can't eat many small meals on a particular day, eat your largest meals in the earlier part of the day. Studies have shown that people lose more weight when they eat their larger meals earlier in the day, while they lose less weight at a slower pace when they eat a larger evening meal.

Be careful about losing too much weight too quickly. Avoid all crash diets, liquid protein diets, extreme diets that are dangerously low in calories, and emotionally depriving diets. These are generally not well-balanced or nutritionally sound. If you have a small frame (ideal weight 100-130 pounds), do not exceed a weight loss of two pounds a week. If you have a larger frame (over 130 pounds), do not lose more than three pounds a week.

Using Artificial Sweeteners to Lose Weight

If you believe that artificial nonnutritive sweeteners will help you lose weight or keep you from becoming overweight, you are in for a surprise. Numerous research studies have shown conclusively that these products have no effect on the amount or level of obesity. According to a February 1987 *Times* article, in a study conducted for the American Cancer Society and published in the *Journal of Preventative Medicine* (March 1986), Steven Stellman and Lawrence Garfinkel found that "women who used artificial sweeteners were more likely to gain weight than women who didn't. They also gained weight faster, regardless of the weight they were to begin with. The researchers surveyed 78,694 women."

This conclusion may apply to aspartame, a newly marketed nonnutritive sweetener found in NutraSweet and Equal. Karen MacNeil, a reporter for *The New York Times*, wrote about a study that was reported in the *Lancet*, the British medical journal (May 1986). According to MacNeil, researchers at Leeds University have concluded that "aspartame may produce a 'residual hunger' that leads to increased food consumption. According to researchers, aspartame may send ambiguous signals to the brain resulting in a loss of control over appetite."

Supplementing Your Diet

Nutritional supplements are important for good nutrition— especially for those trying to lose weight. Nutritional supplements come in many forms. There are vitamins, minerals, amino acids, and special diet products in the form of supplements. Certain nutritional factors such as bioflavonoids, choline, inositol, and various amino acids have been found to assist the body in metabolizing fat more effectively. Let's examine how each of these works in your body.

When you experience a large weight loss, you may also experience bruising of the skin. This bruising results from the loss of padding and mechanical support that had been supplied by the fat to the capillaries. As you reduce body fat through your weight-loss program, bioflavonoid supplementation will help to strengthen your capillaries and prevent this bruising effect. It may take as long as three months to eliminate bruising, even with regular supplementation. In addition to bioflavonoids, you may wish to use choline, a transporter of body fat used as a fuel. Choline works more effectively to reduce fat while increasing energy reserves when it is used together with methionine. If you want to maintain your glucose level during long periods of activity or if you want to control your appetite, inositol can also help.

In addition to these nutritional supplements, the use of amino acids to supplement your diet can help your body eliminate fat. These are available in health food stores or by prescription. Although these amino acids can help some people lose weight, they can easily be abused by someone with a compulsive eating pattern. Even though they may have a well-balanced diet, compulsive eaters still tend to take excessive amounts of amino acids in the belief that more is better. It is strongly recommended that amino acid supplements be used only by those who are on a well-balanced, nutritionally sound weight-loss program.

Some of the amino acids that you might use to supplement your diet include arginine, ornithine, leucine, isoleucine, baline, and methionine. Both arginine and ornithine are nonessential and are known to increase the secretion of HGH (human growth hormone). It is believed that increased HGH triggers the body to burn up fat reserves. Leucine, isoleucine, and baline are used directly by the muscle tissue as a source of energy. It is best to use these amino acids together.

Another amino acid, called carnitine, helps your body use its fat reserves for fuel. It has also been shown to stimulate and maintain the adrenal glands. This subsequently increases your body's use of fat reserves for fuel.

Two other amino acids, D,L phenylalanine and L-tyrosine, function as appetite suppressants and antidepressants. They curb your appetite by releasing chemicals which send messages that you are full to your brain, even if you have not eaten. Phenylalanine may be useful in appetite control by stimulating the secretion of CCK (chaleceptokinin enzyme). L-Tyrosine should be used with vitamin B_6. This vitamin, a natural diuretic that will assist in reducing water weight, is necessary for the action of tyrosine. Before using amino acid supplements, it is important that you confer with your nutritionist or physician in order to learn how to use them safely (some of them do have contraindications).

In addition, arginine and ornithine are two amino acids that stimulate the release of a growth hormone. The release of this growth hormone increases the rate at which your body burns fat and promotes muscle tone.

A good weight-loss program should include each of the following supplements:

- Arginine
- Baline
- Bioflavonoids
- Carnitine
- Choline
- Evening primrose oil
- Inositol
- Isoleucine

- Leucine
- Methionine
- Multiple vitamin-mineral supplement
- Ornithine
- Vitamin B complex
- Vitamin B_6

Juice Therapy

Fresh pressed juices have been used for the last hundred years or so and are among the most recently discovered weight-loss tools. Containing easily absorbed nutrients and plant essences, they have a powerful effect on the body's recuperative powers.

Although juice therapy can be very effective if done under proper supervision, it may be misused by those who are not following a supervised juice therapy program. Many people who overeat will use large amounts of juice in the belief that it is lower in calories than food. Some of these juices may actually contain very high caloric levels without the benefit of fiber. If you are going to use juice therapy for more than a few days, do so under proper supervision.

One sixteen-ounce glass of carrot, beet, or apple juice is recommended daily. Add a teaspoon of bee pollen to this to improve glandular function.

Exercise

Aerobic exercise is very valuable to anyone who is serious about weight control. Exercise increases the rate at which you burn calories not only while you exercise, but for hours afterward. Another benefit of exercise is that your fat is soon replaced with lean muscle tissue. As you gain muscle weight, your body will require more calories. This will enable you to eat more without gaining weight.

A good exercise program provides many benefits for those who wish to reduce or maintain their weight. One advantage of exercise is that an increased number of calories are burned by your body in the hours following an exercise session. This is especially important since the reduced intake of calories while dieting may have actually lowered your body's metabolic rate. Exercise may also help to regulate or even suppress your appetite.

Exercise not only will help you to look and feel fit, but will protect you from disease. Exercising directly reduces your chances of getting the diseases that are most commonly associated with obesity: diabetes, heart disease, and hypertension. You will also look better if you exercise. Since muscle tissue takes up less space than an equal weight of fat tissue, people who exercise regularly look thinner than people who weigh the same but are less sedentary.

Emotional Factors

Of those that I have met who seriously wanted to lose weight, seldom were they able to radically change their eating and exercise patterns in less than five or six months. When a person becomes committed to losing weight, there are many old habits and patterns—both physical and emotional—that have to be altered. This adjustment is seldom easy. Anger, boredom, anxiety, and depression are emotions that often trigger alternating cycles of overeating and tension. By increasing your awareness of how you interact with others, you will be able to address these emotional responses rather than passively watching them arise and becoming victimized by them. A regular program of meditation, visualization, and professional counseling can help you cope with your emotions.

Although there are many factors that determine a person's ability to lose weight, the one factor that is most within your control is the way in which you view life. If you have a poor attitude, you will see everything in this light. If you have an attitude that life is to be lived fully and in celebration, then even the sad and hard times and the times of adversity will not get you down for any longer than it takes for some genuine introspection. In order to successfully lose weight, it is important to have a healing attitude. This is not to be confused with positive thinking. You can certainly choose to view everything positively while it is all collapsing around you; however, this will only be detrimental to the healing process. A healing attitude, on the other hand, involves the ability to perceive all things as possible, even if you do not intellectually understand how this is so. It involves your willingness to perceive yourself as a "healing" organism. Without the strong motivation that comes from your belief that you can change, it will be virtually impossible for you to lose weight and keep it off.

Without strong motivation, it will be extremely difficult to lose weight. By following some suggestions, you may be able to better adapt to your diet. There are a number of support groups available that can help you remain on your weight-loss program. I highly recommend that you join one of these groups so that you can listen to how other dieters handle problems that arise. Overeaters Anonymous has many chapters throughout the United States. Consult your phone book for the center nearest you. Some of their problems may be similar to your own. In these groups, you will hear dieters exchanging their feelings and ideas, as well as their suggestions on how to cope better. Most importantly, these fellow dieters will make you realize that you are not alone.

You can avoid the temptation to eat undesirable foods if you actively resolve to sustain these three conditions: do not make food easily accessible, keep it from full view, and avoid distracting food cues. Eliminating tempting factors will decrease your tendency to overeat. You can create a home environment that is conducive to your weight-loss program. By limiting your access to foods that are not on your program and engaging in activities that focus your attention away from food, you will be in a stronger position to eat well.

How can you control your environment? Ask your friends and family members to avoid bringing food gifts or snacks that will undermine your diet into the house. Build your resistance to commercials about high-calorie foods by watching as few of them as possible. Finally, make eating a wonderful experience in itself. Avoid eating food in association with places, people, or events. Being in these environments may automatically increase your urge to eat high-calorie foods. Learn to be in situations without immediately responding to an urge to eat. Eat only in designated places at specific times.

You will need the support and cooperation of the people around you, so you must make your intentions clear. Be candid when communicating your needs to others. Your firmness will be tested as you make requests of people who tell you that you do not need to lose weight or who attempt to sabotage your weight-loss program. If you are at a party or other social function, friends or new aquaintances may ask why you are not eating certain very high-calorie foods. Explain why you don't want to eat them and do not succumb to any fear of embarrassment that you might have. You *must* be firm. If someone asks you to taste something that they are cooking or eating which would undermine your diet, politely decline. Or if you have ordered food in a restaurant and it is not prepared as you have requested, do not hesitate to have it corrected by speaking with your waiter, waitress, or maitre d'. Finally, try to practice making proper food choices even when you are around others who are eating foods that would ruin your diet.

Food Suggestions

You must decide which foods will provide for a healthy, well-balanced diet. You may have questions about some of your favorites. How much of them is okay? Should you eliminate certain foods from your diet? Are there substitutes for these undesirable foods? What is the best way to prepare your foods? The answers to these questions will help you

determine what changes you should make in order to reduce your fat intake.

What is the best way to prepare your foods? It is better to
broil, bake, steam, or boil your foods than to fry them in oil
or butter. Not only are fried foods hard to digest, but the oil
that breaks down during the frying process may produce
various by-products that are dangerous to your health. See
Chapter 5 for further information on the dangers of frying.
When eating chicken, avoid the fried varieties. When you
prepare vegetables, avoid browning them with meat. (They
act as a fat sponge.) It is also a good idea to refrigerate soup
stocks, stews, and sauces. This will enable you to remove the
hardened surface fat before reheating.

Each of us has our favorite foods—those that we savor
more than all the rest. You will have to decide which foods
you can eliminate from your diet, in favor of ones that are
lower in fat or cholesterol. If you enjoy eating meat, make
sure you trim off any excess fat, choose lean varieties, or replace meat with poultry and fish. If you are going to eat any
animal flesh, it is better to choose poultry, fish, or veal over
beef, pork, or lamb. Use ground round or lean ground beef
instead of regular hamburger or ground chuck. You should
buy leaner cuts of beef rather than the well-marbled cuts.
Try beef bacon, Canadian bacon, or turkey ham instead of
pork bacon.

If you prefer fish, pick those varieties that have a lower oil
content. These include haddock, halibut, flounder, sole, and
tuna that is packed in water rather than oil. Water-packed
tuna has the same content of omega-3 fatty acids as oil-
packed tuna, since the type of oil that tuna is packed in is a
highly processed vegetable oil, not fish oil. (The benefits of
omega-3 fatty acids are discussed in Chapter 4, "The Therapeutic Uses of Oils.") Water-packed tuna should, therefore,
be used instead of oil-packed tuna.

If you are going to eat either meat, poultry, or fish, limit
your portion to no more than two ounces. A side dish of potatoes, brown rice, or whole grain pasta will provide protein
that will balance your meal. Brown rice and whole grain
pasta also contain fiber that can help reduce cholesterol. In-

creasing your intake of fresh fruits, vegetables, and whole grains is always a good idea.

You might want to consider a lacto-vegetarian diet that uses only dairy products prepared from part-skim or nonfat milk. Some tips about dairy products may be helpful. If you enjoy cheese, use skimmed or partially skimmed milk cheese: mozzarella, St. Ortho, or Jarlsburg, for example. These may not be lower in calories, but they do have a lower cholesterol content. Cottage cheese lovers should use low-fat or dry curd cottage cheese instead of creamed cottage cheese. Evaporated skim milk is better for you than evaporated whole milk. And if you use hard cheese, choose those varieties that are made of skim milk. Although these hard cheeses are not very low in fat, they do have less fat, cholesterol, and calories than regular whole milk cheeses. Try to use fewer or smaller amounts of high-fat extras such as margarine, sour cream, cream cheese, mayonnaise, and cream-based salad dressings. I would advise you to limit your intake of butter, cream, and hydrogenated margarine. Instead of margarine or butter, try soy spreads found in health food stores on your bread. Use Neufchâtel cheese rather than cream cheese. If a recipe calls for mayonnaise, use low-fat yogurt or buttermilk, or a low-calorie mayonnaise substitute that contains no cholesterol and is now available in supermarkets. And if you are making quiche or custard, you can add nonfat dry milk powder to liquid milk to prevent a watery mixture.

Some foods should be avoided. In addition to the advice about meats, fish, and dairy products, you should beware of certain foods. For example, you should avoid all fast foods. Most of this type of food is very high in fat. In fact, the palm, palm kernel, and coconut oils that are used in both the preparation of fast food and the manufacture of packaged goods, especially baked goods, are higher in saturated fat than lard. It is wise to avoid processed foods as well. They often contain hidden oils and fats. It is always best to prepare your own food. In this way, you can be sure of what has gone into the meal. If you do eat in a restaurant, ask the waiter or maitre d' which selections are low in fat or not fried. When reading labels, avoid foods that contain partially hardened vegetable oil, hydrogenated vegetable oil, or partially hydrogenated vegetable oil. At buffets, leave the sauce or gravy in the pan. These are usually full of fat and oil. In addition, you should avoid eating foods that are high in refined sugar and starches. These can be converted into saturated fatty acids in the body. Rich desserts, pastries, and candies fall into this category. You can replace these with higher quality foods like fresh peanut butter, nuts, and seeds. (These are still high in fat and should be used in moderation.) It is best to use the raw, roasted, and unsalted varieties of nuts and seeds when eating these foods. For a comparison of the fat and cholesterol content of different foods, refer to Appendix A.

Scientists have known for years that certain vegetable fibers have the ability to bind bile acids, made from cholesterol, which helps you to digest fats and reduce cholesterol levels. New research has shown that calcium pectate, an element found in onions and cabbage, is the element in the fiber most responsible for binding bile acids and lowering cholesterol levels. By following the suggestions mentioned in this chapter, you can reduce the fat content of your meal by 75 percent.

When you begin to alter the types and amounts of fats and oils that you use in your recipes, you will find that the foods on your diet will be just as tasty as before. With some creativity, you can still prepare your favorite recipes by making a few substitutions and changes. It is difficult to eliminate fats and oils totally from cooking since soups, casseroles, stews, and so many others derive much of their flavor from fats. When you reduce the fat level in your cooking, you may wish to compensate for the loss of flavor by adding more seasonings.

Reducing the fat level in recipes may require that you use more liquid to obtain a proper batter consistency. Substituting certain ingredients will reduce the amount of saturated fats in your diet and increase the level of polyunsaturated fats. A decrease in your blood cholesterol level will result from the reduction in saturated fats.

Many people feel that in order to eat healthfully, they have to give up all of the foods that they enjoy. This is not true; however, with a little creativity you can replace those ingredients that are high in fat with those listed below and still enjoy good eating. Try these substitutes:

- Instead of *hydrogenated vegetable shortening,* use the following vegetable oils (listed in order of preference): safflower, sunflower seed, corn, soybean, sesame seed, and cottonseed.

- Instead of using *butter or margarine* when your recipe calls for a hydrogenated or partially hydrogenated vegetable oil, use margarine with a liquid vegetable oil. Margarine is generally made with a hydrogenated or partially hydrogenated vegetable oil.

- When a recipe calls for 1 cup *butter,* use 7/8 cup vegetable oil and 1/2 teaspoon salt instead.

- Instead of using *oil, lard, or butter* to prevent food from sticking in the pan, you can lightly brush liquid lecithin onto the pan. Many nutritionists recommend nonstick skillets, but some natural foods enthusiasts question the safety of the nonstick coating that is used.

- Rather than using *lard or other meat fat, shortening or any other hydrogenated oil, butter, or cocoa butter,* cook with corn oil, safflower oil, sunflower seed oil, sesame seed oil, or soybean oil.

- In place of one ounce (or one square) of *baking chocolate,* use either carob powder or three tablespoons of dry cocoa with one tablespoon of polyunsaturated oil.

- Rather than *cream or creamers made with coconut oil,* try nonfat dry milk.

- Instead of *olive oil,* you can use minced olives to give food an olive oil flavor.

- In place of *frying or sautéing* your food, try baking, steaming, poaching, or broiling it. If you broil, the fat will drip out.

- In place of *whole milk, evaporated whole milk, cream, sour cream, and cream substitutes made with coconut or palm oil,* try either nonfat dry milk, nonfat or skim milk, or evaporated skim milk.

- Instead of *cream cheese and regular whole milk cheese,* use low-fat cottage cheese, farmer cheese, or part-skim ricotta.

- In place of *whole milk or flavored yogurt,* you can add your own flavors to plain low-fat yogurt.

- Rather than using *peanut butter with hydrogenated oil or salted peanuts,* try dried beans, nuts, or unsalted peanuts.

- In place of *regular oil- or mayonnaise-based dressing,* use a salad dressing without an oil base.

- Instead of eating *vegetables in sauce and fruits in syrup,* try fresh fruits, vegetables, and dried fruit.

- Rather than eating *sweetened doughnuts, cookies, and cakes or pancakes, waffles, and muffins that are made from mixes containing hydrogenated fats and oils and white flour,* you should try these: whole grain breads, cracker rolls, flours, pasta, unsweetened whole grain cereals, oatmeal, brown rice, and unrefined corn meal.

- In place of snack foods like *buttered and salted popcorn or salted and roasted nuts and seeds,* try air-popped popcorn or either unroasted or unsalted nuts and seeds.

Avoid Consumption of Refined Carbohydrates

Another factor that can contribute to obesity in addition to leading to other health problems is an overconsumption of refined carbohydrates. Foods containing refined carbohydrates are considered inferior to whole grain products by some nutritionists. The refining process is generally done to increase the shelf life of a product with little concern to the lost nutritional value that occurs during processing. Grain is refined by removing the bran (fiber) and germ of the food, while sugar products are refined by heating and filtering. The most common forms of refined carbohydrates include wheat products (flour, most breakfast meals, pasta, etc.), white rice, and white and brown sugar. During the processing of these foods, many vitamins and minerals are destroyed or filtered out. The loss of vitamins and minerals is a contributing factor to the fat-related disorders that can arise.

When whole grains and unrefined carbohydrates are digested and metabolized, they carry the vitamins and minerals that are essential for these processes to take place. Refined carbohydrates, on the other hand, have been depleted of these essential factors. Thus, when they are metabolized, it is necessary for the body to utilize its own store of nutrients. Many of these essential nutrients are required for the metabolism of fats and cholesterol. If these stores become depleted, the body will have great difficulty converting the excess fats into bile acids and burning off the fat through increased activity. When some of this fat is converted to bile acids, it is eliminated along with cholesterol through the stool.

Excessive consumption of refined carbohydrates can contribute to a long chain of events, beginning with inefficient fat and cholesterol utilization and leading to a decreased rate of metabolism, increased cholesterol levels, and obesity. A decrease in metabolic rate has been associated with various health problems including certain degenerative diseases, certain types of arthritis, cancer, heart disease, and other cardiovascular disorders. Studies show that individuals who are obese have a greater risk of developing cancer, diabetes, and cardiovascular disease. Since certain types of fiber assist the body in removing excess cholesterol, the lack of fiber in refined carbohydrates may contribute to higher cholesterol levels.

ARE ALL CALORIES EQUAL?

A standard line among nutritionists and weight reduction specialists for many years was that "a calorie is the same no matter where you get it from." Recent research, however, now indicates that this may not be the case. A study conducted at the Stanford Center for Research in Disease Prevention lends support to the theory that it is not calories alone that are responsible for weight problems, but rather the composition of the diet itself. In other words, fat calories seem to influence your body in more ways than do calories derived from carbohydrates. The study, which was published in the *American Journal of Clinical Nutrition* and reported in *The New York Times*, was conducted with 155 obese, sedentary men. The study discovered that the fewer the amount of carbohydrates (starches and sugar) and the greater the amount of fat eaten by the men, the greater their percentage of body fat. Neither the number nor the size of the meals that they consumed nor their total caloric intake was related to their percentage of body fat. This research is important because it may help to explain why Americans who consume fewer total calories today are more likely to be overweight than in the past. Although engaging in less activity and exercising less might contribute to weight gain, the actual composition of your diet may also play a significant role. Although it is not yet clear how calories from fat differ from calories from carbohydrates, one explanation for increases in body fat is that they might be related to the body's efficiency in converting ingested fat into body fat. According to an article in *The New York Times*, " . . . only 3 percent of ingested calories are needed to put dietary fat into storage, but converting dietary carbohydrates into body fat uses up 23 percent of the calories consumed."

It is highly unlikely that adults would have a deficiency of fats in their diets, since the amount of essential fatty acids required for good health is quite small. For children, however, the risk of fat deficiency is much greater.

FAT REQUIREMENTS FOR CHILDREN

Many adults assume that tips that help them reduce fat in their diets will also benefit their children. They often believe that their children should drink skim milk and avoid any foods that are high in fat, even those from vegetable sources. Why? These parents feel that they are promoting the health of their children; however, they are misguided. Many parents and educators are concerned that adults are responding to the "eat a low-fat diet" message by putting their children on diets that are too low in calories and fat. Cholesterol and fat are essential for every cell in the body. Without a certain amount of fat, a child cannot grow. A deficiency of cholesterol can even be dangerous for children—especially those under the age of two. Some studies indicate that as many as 25 percent of the infants in the United States under the age of two are on milk that has reduced fat. When a child's diet is deprived of fat, weight gain generally becomes difficult and his rate of growth typically becomes impaired. The child demonstrates an overall inability to thrive. The harmful effects of low-fat diets on children have been supported by a report in the August 1987 issue of *Pediatrics*, the journal of the American Academy of Pediatrics. The study found that children were often placed on low-fat diets by parents who were following guidelines established for adults in order to reduce their risk of cardiovascular disease. Doctors cited in the study found that when these babies were put on balanced diets with a greater fat intake, they gained weight and began to grow.

Children under two years of age require more fat for growth than they do for any other period in their lives. Growth is very rapid in the first two years of life. Essential fats are still developing in the central nervous system at this age. Infants and toddlers require a large intake of calories, and fats are its most concentrated source. Although there are many areas of controversy among physicians and nutritionists concerning dietary fat levels in adult diets, no such controversy exists concerning the fat intake of children.

It is best for young children to be breast-fed, unless it is impossible for some medical reason. If breastfeeding is not an option, then a well-balanced formula should be substituted as the source of nutrition. Both breast milk and commercial formula both contain twenty calories per ounce. Breast milk is 52 percent fat while formula is required to have at least 30 to 54 percent fat.

While medical doctors generally recommend that a baby be weaned from breast milk to formula or from formula to whole cow's milk, the trend among many nutritionists is now away from this due to the belief that cow's milk may contribute to various allergies when fed to children. Whole goat's milk is an alternative, as are cultured whole milk products such as yogurt and kefir. The child, however, should *not* be weaned onto low-fat or skim milk products.

It is important for young children to avoid low-fat diets; however, if your child comes from a family with a history of heart disease, consult your physician. In such cases, it may be advisable to place the child on a low-fat, low-cholesterol diet. In order to determine if this is necessary, have your child tested for serum cholesterol before the age of two if your family's medical history indicates high cholesterol levels and coronary artery disease. Even if your family history does not indicate any risk, you can have your child's cholesterol levels checked after the age of four or five. This evaluation may not be necessary if the child is from a vegetarian family.

There is currently no consensus concerning the optimal percentage of fat for children over two years of age. In fact, a number of respected medical and research groups have greatly differing points of view on this issue. Many pediatricians claim that there has been no evidence for reducing the level of calories derived from fat to less than 30 to 40 percent of the total diet. A report in the September 1986 issue of the journal of the American Academy of Pediatrics states, "Any recommendations for changing towards a more restrictive dietary pattern during the first two decades of life should await demonstration that such dietary restrictions would support adequate growth and development for children and adolescents." On the other hand, a number of groups including the American Health Foundation, the American Heart Association, and a panel sponsored by the National Institutes of Health recommend that diets for children be more restrictive concerning fats. They recommend that fat intake be no more than 30 percent of the total diet.

Because of these differing points of view on how much fat to allow your child after the age of two, you may be confused about what to include in your child's diet. There are some things you *can* do to insure a healthy diet. Make sure that your child avoids fried and junk foods. Including plenty of fresh fruits and vegetables is always a good idea, and I would advise that your child eat raw rather than roasted nuts and seeds. Make sure that you include plenty of whole grain foods as well as moderate amounts of dairy foods and naturally processed oils in your child's diet.

Designing a diet that meets your needs based upon your age, sex, and body size is important for good health. The suggestions offered in this chapter were designed to help you meet your dietary goals. Not only are fats and oils essential elements of a well-balanced diet, but they also have therapeutic uses. The next chapter discusses the benefits of certain oils for various disorders and explains how to use them most effectively.

4
Therapeutic Uses
of Oils

In addition to the many roles that fats and oils play as essential nutrients, there are many oils that are valued for their therapeutic and healing qualities. Studies reveal that the use of certain oils helps to lower cholesterol and triglyceride levels and blood pressure; to relieve pain associated with migraines, arthritis, joint inflammation, and other injuries; and to promote skin tone and healthy hair. Some of these oils, like evening primrose oil and castor oil, are derived from herbs, while others like cod-liver oil are derived from animal sources. All therapeutic oils are commonly used as healing agents rather than as basic nutrients.

BENEFITS OF GAMMA LINOLENIC ACID
(EVENING PRIMROSE OIL)

There is a "wonder substance" that, according to some experts, is likely to become extremely popular—perhaps even more so than vitamin C. This substance is gamma linolenic acid (also called GLA or evening primrose oil).

GLA has been called the "wonder substance" because research has shown it to be beneficial in producing positive results with so many different ailments. Among the benefits associated with GLA are that it:

- Induces weight loss in persons who are 10 percent or more over their ideal weight without dieting. (It does not affect the weight of those persons of normal weight.)
- Prevents withdrawal symptoms and lessens the craving for alcohol in alcoholics.
- Lowers cholesterol levels and blood pressure.
- Inhibits the formation of blood clots.
- Alleviates symptoms associated with diseases of the kidneys, eyes, and heart in diabetics.
- Normalizes the composition of essential fatty acids in patients suffering from multiple sclerosis, and can possibly stabilize their condition.
- Helps to alleviate schizophrenia, manic depression, ulcers, hypertension, dysmenorrhea, arthritis, and premenstrual syndrome.

Sources of GLA in substantial amounts are very limited; breast milk and a few botanical sources, such as evening primrose oil and black currant seed, are the major ones. Gamma linolenic acid, an intermediate fatty acid, is essential for the body to produce the all-important prostaglandins PG_1 and PG_2. GLA may be converted from linoleic acid in your body; however, there are many inhibitors to this conversion. As a result, it is recommended by some nutritionists that GLA be included directly in the diet.

BENEFITS OF OMEGA-3 FATTY ACIDS

In the mid-1980s, many magazines and newspapers reported on the newly discovered health benefits derived from the oils of certain plants and cold-water, deep-sea fish. Because these oils were an integral part of the Eskimos' diets, interest in them was stimulated when it was found that Eskimos had extremely low levels of heart disease despite diets that were high in fat. These oils contain what are known as omega-3 fatty acids, and are found primarily in bluefish, salmon, sardines, and tuna (including canned varieties of tuna and salmon).

Fish Sources

You will not receive high levels of omega-3 fatty acids simply by eating fish. You may eat a four-ounce serving of cod, a low-fat fish, and receive only 300 milligrams of omega 3s, while a similar serving of salmon can contain 3,600 milligrams of omega 3s. To find out which types of fish contain the highest amounts of omega-3 fatty acids, refer to Appendix A. Omega-3 fatty acids largely consist of two components: EPA (eicosapentaenoic acid) and DHA (docosahexaeoic acid). Preliminary studies have shown that omega-3 fatty acids seem to reduce cholesterol levels and inhibit blood clotting as well. Some researchers remain skeptical about the therapeutic effects of fish oils. They question whether reduced cholesterol and clotting results from the fish oils themselves or rather from a decreased consumption of meat and other foods that are high in fat. Despite these criticisms, it has been shown that your level of LDLs (low-density lipoproteins, which are a bad form of cholesterol) will increase when your intake of fish oils is reduced. In fact, even low dosages of fish oil will reduce triglyceride levels.

Some of the health benefits associated with omega-3 fatty acids are:

- Reduced risk of atherosclerosis, a disease in which hardening of the arteries occurs.
- Decreased risk of heart disease.
- Minimized formation of blood clots.
- Lowered blood cholesterol and triglyceride levels.
- Reduced risk of high blood pressure.

Fish Oil Supplementation

Some people will choose fish oil supplementation rather than fish to increase their intake of omega-3 fatty acids because they either dislike the taste of fish or wish to avoid too high an intake of oil in their diets. Unfortunately, those fish that have high levels of omega-3 fatty acids also tend to contain large amounts of fat. In addition, some of these fish may be high in cholesterol or may live in polluted waters containing mercury, cadmium, PCBs, or other toxic agents. These concerns were voiced in a letter addressed to the editor of *The New York Times* by Grant Higginson, M.D. (Maternity Services and Family Planning), Diane St. Clair (Pregnancy Healthline), and Alan Stern (Chief, Division of Environmental Toxicology, New York City Department of Health). The letter appearing in *The New York Times* (September 18, 1985) states, in part, that ". . . the New York State Department of Environmental Conservation suggests that, as a general guideline, persons consume no more than one fish meal per week from inland waters of New York State." The department further advises that "high-risk groups such as pregnant women, breast-feeding mothers, and young children refrain completely from eating certain species of fish from specific New York State waters." The letter also points out that "both human and animal research suggests that PCB's . . . may cause nervous system disorders and other adverse effects when consumed in contaminated foods."

Certain fish oil supplements will state on their labels that the source of their fish oil has been shown to be contaminant free as well as cholesterol free. When buying fish oil capsules, be sure to choose a brand that contains an antioxidant from a natural source. The antioxidant will prevent the oils from becoming rancid.

Many nutritionists and physicians feel that using foods that are high in omega-3 fatty acids or using non-fish sources for the nutrient is a better and safer approach than using unregulated dosages of fish oil capsules.

Alternatives to Fish Oil for Omega-3 Fatty Acids

Although many of the studies citing the benefits of omega-3 fatty acids were conducted with fish oils, there are alternative sources for these important fatty acids. The best source of omega-3 fatty acids, containing more omega 3 than fish, is fresh flax oil. Omega-3 fatty acids derived from flax oil are probably a better choice than those derived from fish. They generally do not have free radicals, pesticides, trans-fatty acids, or PCBs. Flax oil also costs less than fish oil.

BENEFICIAL EFFECTS OF FISH OIL

In addition to containing omega-3 fatty acids, fish oils have been shown to have beneficial effects on patients suffering from migraines, rheumatoid arthritis, other forms of arthritis, and high cholesterol levels.

Effects of Fish Oil on Migraines

Recent preliminary studies have shown that a fatty acid which is found in fish oil, EPA (eicosapentaenoic acid), may have some benefits in the treatment of headaches. One study consisted of volunteers who had suffered from severe migraine headaches that were unrelieved by drugs. These individuals experienced a marked improvement when they took fish oil capsules that were equivalent to eating seven ounces of fish each day. The study also found that the clients who had the greatest relief from pain also had the highest levels of EPA in their red blood cell membranes. In a previous study, EPA levels in these same cells were found to be lower in those individuals who had the most severe migraines. According to Dr. Charles J. Glueck, director of the General Clinical Research Center and the Lipid Research Clinic at the University of Cincinnati College of Medicine, the effects of EPA may result from its reduction of serotonin in the body and its influence on the metabolic rate of prostaglandin. Both of these natural body substances have an important role in the development of migraine headaches.

Effects of Fish Oil on Rheumatoid Arthritis

EPA has also produced some positive results in patients afflicted with moderate types of rheumatoid arthritis. In studies conducted in New York and Boston, participants who took fish oil capsules equivalent to 7–9 ounces of fish oil in addition to their usual medications experienced less inflammation and joint tenderness. Since this was a preliminary study, however, it was felt that more research would be necessary before any conclusive evidence could be indicated in favor of fish oil supplementation for patients with rheumatoid arthritis.

Research conducted at Harvard University by Dr. Richard Sperling and other researchers revealed that the addition of fish oil to the diets of two groups of patients, one stricken with arthritis and the other without inflammatory disease, produced similar results in the blood cells as in the previous study. These results were due to a shift from production of a highly inflammatory substance, leukotriene B_4, to production of the much less inflammatory leukotriene B_5. During the test period the inflamed patients reported feeling less pain and tenderness in the joints.

Effects of Cod-Liver Oil on Arthritis and High Cholesterol

As early as 1770, cod-liver oil was recognized as a valuable supplement for the elderly and sickly. Then, in 1822, this fish oil was used to treat rickets, although it was not until 1921 that cod-liver oil was viewed as a specific remedy for this condition.

In the last thirty years, Dale Alexander, a lay author, has greatly publicized the value of cod-liver oil in relieving some of the symptoms of arthritis. Although medical researchers have dismissed his controversial claims as quackery, many people have come to agree with and support Alexander's contention that this oil creates a visibly profound reduction of arthritic symptoms.

Among the benefits associated with cod-liver oil are that it:

• Enhances the general health of the skin, including its softness.

• Enhances the tone and lustre of hair.

- Demonstrates bactericidal and bacteriostatic properties.

- Is a good source of vitamin D.

- Promotes increased utilization of calcium, most probably due to its vitamin D content.

- Reduces cholesterol levels. This may be due to the lecithin, arachidonic acid, vitamin D, or other naturally occurring factors found in cod-liver oil.

- Is a rich source of unsaturated fatty acids, iodine, bromine, and other trace minerals.

- Contains vitamin A and vitamin D in a 10-to-1 ratio, which is higher than any other source found in nature.

Even though cod-liver oil was a popular remedy, its disagreeable taste and odor made it difficult to use regularly. In an attempt to make the oil more palatable, manufacturers have in recent years begun packaging the oil in capsule form and offering mint- and cherry-flavored cod-liver oil in liquid form.

BENEFITS OF AROMA THERAPY

The use of oils that are derived from plants, generally called aromatic oils or essences, as healing agents is an ancient practice that seems to have crossed all boundaries of time and culture. These essences are used for physical ailments as well as for the treatment of psychological disorders, and are an important part of any health-building program. Although a number of essences are produced synthetically, there is a strong feeling among healers and physicians who work with them as therapeutic tools that the results obtainable with the synthetic product cannot compare with those obtained from the essence derived from a plant.

According to Jean Valnet, a respected authority on the subject, "Aromatic essences are volatile, oily, fragrant and generally colorless substances which can be obtained from plants." Aroma therapy is different from any other form of natural therapy in that essential oils can act on many levels:

the physical level, the energy level, the emotional level, and the psychic level. Using aromatic oils can be simple at the same time that they can be complex. They can be used both therapeutically, as part of your beauty care routine, and as perfume.

Essences may be extracted from plants by a variety of methods including distillation, pressing, tapping, and heating, and through the use of various solvents. After the essences have been extracted from the plant, they can be administered in a variety of ways: through inhalation or applied compresses, orally, by massaging specific body parts with them, or by adding them to your bath water. Although essences may be used individually, they are often used in combination. Many of these are not pleasing when used alone, but in combination they can create a very pleasant scent.

Two factors are most important in the use of plant essences: the pure quality and the proper dosage, since they are extremely powerful and can even be poisonous if used improperly or in too high a dosage. In healing illnesses of the nervous system, "stimulating oils," such as the oils of cardamon, cedar, cinnamon, fennel, lemon, and ylang-ylang, might be used. These are particularly effective in addressing the lack of nerve function that is typical of certain types of paralysis and voice loss. More "sedating oils," such as cajuput, camomile, Melissa, and peppermint, might be used for relieving insomnia and extreme nervousness.

HOW TO USE AROMA THERAPY

Aroma therapy involves simple techniques. In fact, merely opening a bottle of aromatic plant oils will fill the room with an aroma in a short time. Most aroma therapists use these oils for specific purposes. They will generally use a specific technique in order to obtain the healing benefits of essential oils for their clients.

Essential oils can be dispersed effectively in a room by means of a fine aerosal spray. In this way, the antiseptic and healing qualities are made available. Some antiseptic essences include the oils of lemon, thyme, orange, bergamot, juniper, clove, citronella, lavender, niaouli, peppermint, rosemary, sandalwood, and eucalyptus. Some people may be allergic or sensitive to some component of the spray. For these individuals a simple and acceptable way to obtain the benefits of inhaling the healing essence is to purchase a small heat lamp with a crucible above it. You may put several drops of the essence into the crucible, and the heat will naturally disperse it. Such lamps are usually available from companies that distribute essential oils and essences.

Another way to use plant oils is topically. Since many essences are extremely concentrated, the best way of applying them is to soak compresses in diluted essences and apply them twice daily. You may also use plant oils as a healing agent by applying them on your chest using friction. You should mix the essences in a base of lanolin and cocoa butter, and then rub on the chest once in the morning and once at night.

You may also use these oils orally. Using no more than four or five essences in combination, place 25–40 drops (limiting each oil to about 8 drops) in a glass of lukewarm water. Take three times daily, ten minutes before meals. A child's dosage should be limited to 3–10 drops three times daily. (When placed in hot water, essences tend to evaporate quickly. Since some essences are too powerful to be taken orally, this practice should be done with caution.)

THERAPEUTIC EFFECTS OF MASSAGING OILS

For thousands of years, oils have been used to massage the skin. They serve to lubricate and heal the skin using touch. It is believed that different oils can rid your body of toxins through the skin and demonstrate their healing capabilities in your body. Moisturizers and other skin-care products derive their soothing emollient effect from the oils that are used in their preparation. Although mineral oil is the primary ingredient of most cosmetics, manufacturers of natural massage oil and skin cream use natural oils such as avocado, sweet almond, wheat germ, and peanut oil. Many natural healers and massage therapists feel that it is best to avoid mineral oil, since this petroleum derivative can draw the fat-soluble vitamins from the skin and dry it with long-term use. There are other hypoallergenic oils available that are equally as effective.

THERAPEUTIC USES OF CASTOR OIL

This oil is derived from the castor bean. Although eating the bean itself would be toxic, the oil can be used safely in small doses. At one time castor oil was a home remedy for constipation; however, it is seldom used for this purpose any longer. Although this oil has traditionally been used as a laxative, it is not recommended for this purpose. Approximately 80 percent of the fatty acid content of castor oil is made of ricinoleic acid, a hydroxyl fatty acid that acts as a laxative. Constant internal use of castor oil may result in a loss of essential vitamins and minerals from the intestinal tract, and may cause nutritional deficiencies and laxative dependence.

Castor oil is commonly used in natural healing. Compresses and herbal packs are applied to help heal injuries and joint inflammations.

Not all fats and oils are beneficial. You have read about the positive nutritional benefits of evening primrose oil, gamma linolenic acid, and omega-3 fatty acids, and about the healing effects of aroma therapy and castor oil. There are, however, many health problems associated with a large intake of "bad" fats. The following chapter will help you identify which fats can be detrimental to your health. You will then be able to reduce your consumption of the "bad" fats, while still enjoying the nutritional value of the "good" fats.

5
Understanding and Reducing the Dangers of Fats and Oils

Americans love fat. We love it so much that 40 percent of our caloric intake is derived from this substance. That's about 10 percent more than is healthy, and we are paying a great price for it. Many Americans recognize that reducing their fat intake will prevent or lessen obesity; however, what they fail to realize is that it will eliminate other health problems as well. By cutting down your total fat intake, you can avoid the health problems associated with increased fat intake including hyperlipemia, high triglyceride levels, cancer, hypertension, and hearing loss.

In the last eighty years, statistics have shown a great increase in diseases associated with fatty degeneration. The death rate resulting from cardiovascular disease in 1900 comprised only 15 percent of all deaths. Today that rate has risen by 350 percent. Cardiovascular disease now accounts for almost 50 percent of all deaths. The number of deaths due to cancer, liver degeneration, diabetes, multiple sclerosis, and kidney degeneration has also increased.

Fat is so much a part of our food culture that we aren't even aware of it. Can you imagine eating salad without salad dressing? How many people do you know that eat pasta salad, egg salad, potato salad, or tuna salad without mayonnaise? Man may not live by bread alone, but few people eat bread alone—they usually put something with lots of fat on it. This may take the form of butter, margarine, or peanut butter, but it is high in fat just the same.

One of the greatest disadvantages of fats is that they have approximately 250 calories per ounce. That is about 40 calories per teaspoon of fat. This amount is more than twice that contained in an equivalent amount of protein or carbohydrate. You are more likely to overeat with foods containing fat than you would with foods containing protein or carbohydrates since fats are low in bulk. It is obviously easier to eat one doughnut than it would be to eat two heads of iceburg lettuce, yet they are of equal caloric value. Actually, if you think about it, it is probably easier to eat four doughnuts than two entire heads of iceburg lettuce. I think you get the picture. You can refer to Chapter 3 for tips on how to reduce unnecessary fat from your diet.

There are no fats that are totally unsaturated or saturated. All fats have a combination of fatty acids. When you hear that a certain fat is saturated, what is actually meant is that it has a predominant amount of saturated fatty acids. This is true about butter. Consequently, a food will be identified as a result of its monosaturated and polyunsaturated fats because these types of fatty acids predominate in the food; however, a food containing them will contain some saturated fats as well.

PRITIKIN'S VIEWS ON HIGH FAT LEVELS

The Pritikin program is a nutrition and lifestyle plan developed a number of years ago by Nathan Pritikin. Even though it was initially viewed as "this year's fad diet," the program became very popular for its clarity of thought and sensible suggestions and for the support it received from many nutritionists and physicians. Pritikin's program is based on his belief that high fat levels damage the body. Until Pritikin presented his views, many people felt that saturated fats were dangerous to the body and that a diet high in polyunsaturates was very safe and healthy. Pritikin's program indicated that the healthiest diet would be one that allows *no more than 5 to 10 percent fat*, and claimed that many health authorities were still recommending that diets be no more than 30 percent fat despite evidence supporting Pritikin's position.

According to Pritikin, fats can damage your body in the following three ways:

1. They suffocate your tissues by depriving them of the necessary oxygen.

2. They raise the levels of uric acid and cholesterol in your tissues. (High cholesterol levels have been shown to contribute to gout and atherosclerosis.)

3. They interfere with carbohydrate metabolism, which may contribute to maturity onset diabetes.

Pritikin also asserted that regardless of whether fats were of animal or vegetable origin, they tend to surround the formed elements of the blood—especially the red blood cells and platelets—with a fatty film. This fatty film causes the blood elements to clump and stick together, plugging up blood vessels and capillaries in such a way that up to 20 percent of your blood flow is obstructed. If you happen to smoke, the oxygen tie-up that results from this habit in combination with a high-fat diet will aggravate the situation and reduce circulation even more.

Pritikin recommends that you avoid an intake of fats other than those that are naturally occurring in your diet. Pritikin applauds those who are vegetarian, yet has some recommendations for those who feel that this type of diet is too restrictive. He advises that you eat plenty of fruits, vegetables, grains, and, if necessary, lean chicken and fish. He suggests that you avoid whole milk products, meat, eggs, oils, oil-based salad dressings, nuts, and seeds.

Pritikin's diet is generally considered excellent by most nutritionists because it helps to avoid clogged arteries and heart disease. As respected as Pritikin's program is, however, it does have its limitations. For example, Pritikin does not recognize that certain foods having a high fat content, like omega-3 fatty acids, and soy foods may help to lower cholesterol levels. Pritikin may simply have been unaware of the studies conducted in various Italian medical centers by C.R. Sirtori. Dr. Sirtori worked with individuals having very high cholesterol levels who were unable to reduce their cholesterol levels by eating low-fat diets. After Dr. Sirtori gave soy foods to these individuals, their cholesterol levels quickly dropped within the normal range. Pritikin also ignores what is called the pyridoxine-methionine theory, which discusses nutritional factors other than cholesterol when reviewing the epidemiological data on heart disease.

Another limitation of Pritikin's program is its exclusion of nutritional supplementation. Pritikin feels supplementation is unnecessary. Like many others, Pritikin believes that you can get all of the vitamins and minerals that you require by eating a well-balanced, healthy diet. Many studies have shown the health benefits of various supplements. Stress, along with the constant health threat posed by poor air and water quality, seems to warrant a basic supplementation program.

Before you can create a well-balanced dietary program, you must be aware of the risks associated with certain types and amounts of fats and oils and the dangers associated with heating these nutrients to high temperatures and exposing them to oxygen during their manufacture, processing, and use.

UNDERSTANDING CHOLESTEROL

It seems that almost every week new information adds to the cholesterol controversy. Mention that a particular food product contains cholesterol, and people immediately form mental images of clogged arteries and heart attacks. Many people have been confused by all of the negative publicity surrounding cholesterol in recent years. First, you've heard that cholesterol is bad for you. Recently you may have heard about good cholesterol. What does it all mean?

As mentioned in Chapter 2, cholesterol is a waxy substance that is closely related to the adrenal and sex hormones. Eggs, poultry, meat, fish, shellfish, and other animal foods contain various amounts of cholesterol.

Unlike the essential fatty acids, which must be obtained from your diet, cholesterol can be manufactured by the body. Your cells will manufacture cholesterol from the by-products of protein, fat, and carbohydrate digestion as it is needed in the body. For example, cholesterol will be manufactured in the placenta of pregnant women. It is needed during pregnancy to produce progesterone, a hormone that keeps the pregnancy from terminating.

Health problems arise when your diet is high in fat, especially saturated or other nonessential fatty acids. Excess fat is converted to cholesterol in the body. In the average human body there are about 150,000 milligrams of cholesterol, 700 milligrams of which are carried in the blood. The amount of cholesterol in your body will vary according to your health, body size, and dietary program.

Approximately 50 percent of the cholesterol obtained from the diet is not absorbed or used by the body. The other 50 percent is used to perform essential functions or may contribute to a number of health problems. Because the body converts excess fat to cholesterol, individuals who have a high fat or sugar intake tend to have greater cholesterol levels than people who eat less of these compounds in their diets.

Cholesterol can be carried in the blood by any of three lipoproteins: high-density lipoproteins (HDLs), low-density lipoproteins (LDLs), and very-low-density lipoproteins (VLDLs). The type of lipoprotein that carries the cholesterol affects how it will be used by the body and whether it will be beneficial or detrimental to your health. High LDL and VLDL levels can contribute to the accumulation of cholesterol plaques in the arteries, which is a major factor in cardiovascular disease.

Research studies conducted in Finland have shown that each 1 percent decrease of LDL levels in your blood lowers your risk of heart disease by 2 percent. These studies have also indicated that increasing your level of HDLs leads to a decreased risk of heart disease. This study, which was published in the November 1987 issue of *The New England Journal of Medicine*, used complex statistical analysis and was able to eliminate all other factors that might contribute to heart disease from the study except for cholesterol.

In a November 1983 article from *Time* magazine, Antonio Gotto, a cholesterol expert from the Baylor College of Medicine in Houston, says, "The garden-variety person with cardiovascular disease, maybe 60% of heart attack patients, has a low HDL level and only a moderately high LDL level. Changing HDL levels will be very important for them." These revealing statistics have helped nutritional researchers understand why cholesterol poses a health risk in some people, while it promotes good health in others. They discovered that high-density lipoproteins not only are safe, but actually help the body get rid of cholesterol. The Finnish study clearly indicates that raising low levels of HDL and lowering high levels of LDL is an effective approach to reducing the risk of heart disease.

Cholesterol levels are measured in milligrams per deciliter (mg/dl). The concentration of cholesterol in the blood is determined by measuring the weight of cholesterol (in milligrams) in one deciliter of blood. Figure 5.1 depicts the ratio of serum cholesterol to high-density lipoprotein. This ratio is calculated by taking the total cholesterol count and dividing it by the HDL level. Thus, if you have a total cholesterol level of 200 milligrams per deciliter and an HDL level of 40 milligrams per deciliter, the ratio of total cholesterol to HDL would be 5.0. The higher the ratio of total cholesterol to HDL, the greater the risk of heart disease.

Despite the negative publicity often received by cholesterol, there are many bodily functions that could not take place without it. See Chapter 2 for the many essential functions that cholesterol performs in the body. Discussion of cholesterol in this chapter, however, will be limited to reducing the dangers of "bad" cholesterol while maintaining the proper amounts of "good" cholesterol.

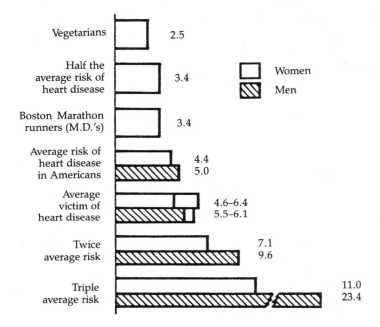

Figure 5.1   Ratio of Serum Cholesterol to HDL

Source: *HDL Cholesterol, A Technical Monograph.* Published by National Health Laboratories, Inc. 1987. Reprinted with permission.

THE EFFECTS OF FAT INTAKE
ON CHOLESTEROL LEVELS

Although cholesterol itself is not a fat, cholesterol levels in the body are greatly affected by fat. When people discuss dietary fat, cholesterol is usually a part of the conversation as well.

Many people do not understand the differences between fat and cholesterol. In recent years people have become more aware of the health risks attributed to certain types of cholesterol and have begun to modify their eating habits. Since the mid-1960s, many people have increased their intake of poultry and fish and have greatly decreased their use of red meat and eggs. Instead of ordering high-fat foods like beef- and pork-based deli meats (salami, bologna, sausage), many people are now purchasing those made from turkey and chicken, which generally have a lower fat content.

It has become clear that it is not just the amount of cholesterol in your diet that will affect blood cholesterol levels, but also the type and amount of fat that you consume. In fact, evidence seems to indicate that your total fat intake will have an even greater effect on blood cholesterol than the amount of cholesterol in your diet. This might explain why some people choose veal over beef. Even though veal has a higher cholesterol content ounce for ounce than beef, it is much lower in fat than beef. Some physicians recommend that you eat veal rather than beef to lower cholesterol. This does not mean that you should begin using large amounts of polyunsaturated fat either, for while it is true that they can reduce your levels of LDL and VLDL cholesterol (the undesirable lipoproteins) in the blood, they can also reduce HDL cholesterol (the desirable lipoprotein). Monounsaturated fats like olive oil are most desirable because they reduce the levels of LDLs and VLDLs without affecting HDLs.

RISKS ASSOCIATED WITH HIGH FAT LEVELS

There are many dangers associated with consumption of a diet high in fat, especially since excess fat is converted to cholesterol. Among the many health problems associated with high fat levels are coronary heart disease, hyperlipemia, cancer, hypertension, and hearing loss.

Coronary Heart Disease

If you have high fat and blood cholesterol levels, you increase your risk of suffering a heart attack. A new theory was published recently in *The New York Times* in an attempt to explain why this happens. The October 1988 article states, "When plaques build up inside the coronary arteries, the flow of oxygen-rich blood to the heart can be impeded causing chest pain and leaving the patient vulnerable to complete blockage by a blood clot and thus a life threatening heart attack." This theory suggests that cholesterol will not form plaques unless it has been oxidized. Thus, if the oxidation of cholesterol can be prevented, so can the formation of plaques, according to Dr. Guy M. Chislom of The Cleveland Clinic Foundation, a leading heart institute. Avoiding oxidized cholesterol and its resulting plaque is important to cardiovascular health. When your blood becomes overloaded with these substances, they begin to build up along the circulatory plumbing, particularly the arteries of the brain and heart. Over time your arteries may become narrower and clogged. This plaque formation, along with the narrowing of these important arteries, forces your heart to pump harder to deliver vital oxygen and nutrients throughout your body. A clot formation can entirely close the blood's passageway. When one of the main vessels to the heart becomes blocked, the result is a **heart attack**.

A **stroke** results when the arteries of the brain are blocked. Other factors besides a diet high in fats and cholesterol, such as high blood pressure and cigarette smoking, can also increase your risk of heart attack; however, consuming large amounts of fats and cholesterol has been shown to be a health risk.

Populations like ours with diets high in saturated fats and cholesterol tend to have high blood cholesterol levels. Individuals within these populations usually have greater risks of having heart attacks than people with diets low in fat and cholesterol. Eating an increased amount of saturated fat and cholesterol will increase blood cholesterol levels in most people; however, this will vary according to genetic factors and the way in which your body uses cholesterol. Some people can consume diets high in saturated fats and cholesterol and still maintain normal blood cholesterol levels. Other less fortunate people have high blood cholesterol levels even though they eat low-fat, low-cholesterol diets.

It seems as if there has always been a controversy of one sort or another over all these low-fat, low-cholesterol warnings. Are these dietary recommendations really necessary for healthy Americans? The consensus among most experts is that the United States population as a whole needs to reduce its current intake of total fat, saturated fat, and cholesterol. This suggestion is especially appropriate for people who have high blood pressure or who smoke.

Hyperlipemia

As more information is gathered on the good and bad lipids, researchers can more easily identify and treat disorders of blood lipids. An entire family of disorders caused by hyperlipemia (excessive fat in the blood) has been identified. These conditions vary based on their cause, the types of lipids involved, and their response to treatment. There are seldom any outward signs of hyperlipemia. People with this condition will sometimes have small bumps on certain parts of their body, particularly the hands, eyelids, elbows, heels, and knees. These bumps, which may be unattractive as well as uncomfortable, are composed of fatty substances deposited in the tissues. Some hyperlipemic patients will experience abdominal pains, but this is uncommon.

Therefore, if your diet is too high in fat, you are more at risk to certain dangers—some that are apparent and some that are not so obvious. Even though the symptoms of hyperlipemia are not obvious, you should be aware of this condition. Although there are many causes for this condition, many physicians believe that the most important ones are poor eating habits, lack of exercise, and heredity. It is important to keep in mind that eating saturated fats does not lead to this disorder; it arises from total fat intake. Although replacing saturated fats with polyunsaturated fats will reduce your risk of cardiovascular and heart disease, using large amounts of polyunsaturated fats may increase the formation of free radicals in your body (discussed later in this chapter) and increase your risk of cancer.

Physicians have acknowledged that genetics can play a role in hyperlipemia. If you have this condition, chances are very good that one or more of your family members has it as well. Often a physician will examine you for this condition based on the fact that one of your family members has the condition.

The types of food you eat may influence the form your hyperlipemia takes. For example, one form of this condition is characterized by an excessively high cholesterol level. In such a situation, eating too many fatty meats, rich dairy products, and other foods that increase blood cholesterol levels is best avoided.

If, on the other hand, your condition is characterized by high levels of triglycerides, then you may be eating excessive amounts of sweet and starchy foods. Why two people with the same exact diet may not both be susceptible to hyperlipemia is still a mystery, but it does happen.

Although high fat intake is generally associated with hyperlipemia, if it is characterized by high triglyceride levels, then eating starches (especially pasta made from white flour), bread, desserts, white rice, or other refined carbohydrates will only aggravate the condition. It is also important to reduce or eliminate your use of alcohol. Individuals with high triglyceride levels tend also to be overweight, so any dietary program should take into consideration calorie control as well as triglyceride reduction.

Cancer

Various studies indicate that there is a strong association between the total dietary fat intake and the rate of breast cancer. Although it is unclear what the connection is between a high fat intake and breast cancer, many researchers believe that it may be hormonal. When you eat foods containing fat, hormone production is stimulated in your body. Some scientists believe that abnormal levels of prolactin, androgens, and estrogen may put excessive stress on breast tissue cells. It is believed that this stress eventually leads to breast cancer. A study examining the changes in hormone levels that occur due to a greater fat intake tends to support the connection between high fat intake and breast cancer. The results of this particular study were published in 1979 in *Federation Proceedings*.

After compiling the breast cancer rates in forty-one countries, G. Hems of the Department of Community Medicine in Aberdeen, Scotland, was able to show that "variation of breast cancer rates between countries arose predominately from differences in diet." The mortality rates from breast cancer for Seventh-day Adventists are one-half to two-thirds that of Americans in general. This may very well be due to the fact that many Adventists are on low-fat or vegetarian diets. Studies of Japanese immigrants also indicate a correlation between a high fat intake and cancer. When the Japanese immigrants replaced their low-fat diets with diets high in fat, their rate of bowel cancer increased.

Evidence suggests that increased fat in the diet leads not only to increased cancer rates, but also to increased incidence of cardiovascular disease. Studies sponsored by the American Heart Association indicate a correlation between the levels and types of fat that we consume and our probability of experiencing a heart attack or stroke or other cardiovascular problems.

Hypertension

Controlled research studies conducted by the United States Department of Agriculture have shown that when the diet is high in polyunsaturated fats, there is a reduction in elevated blood pressure levels in adults. Thus, if you follow the recommendations to lower cholesterol levels, there is a good chance that you will lower your blood pressure as well. This is a healthy way to reduce two major risk factors for heart disease.

Hearing Loss

Research indicates that much of the hearing loss in the United States that we associate with aging is actually a result of atherosclerosis. In atherosclerosis, cholesterol deposits build up in the arteries that supply the ear as well as the rest of your body.

A number of studies have indicated that when someone with a hearing problem due to atherosclerosis switches to a low-fat diet, hearing loss can be stopped and even reversed. A long-term Finnish study placed 4,000 individuals on low-fat diets for six years. These individuals not only had fewer heart attacks, but also had superior acuity than those who continued to eat a diet high in fat. An October 1985 article in *The New York Times* reported that "when the diets of the two groups were reversed, the group now on the high-fat diet experienced hearing losses, while hearing improved in the low-fat diet group."

BENEFITS OF CUTTING DOWN ON TOTAL FAT INTAKE AND CHOLESTEROL

If you reduce the amount of fat in your diet, you will experience many benefits. Because all types of fat, both saturated and polyunsaturated, are the most concentrated source of calories when compared with proteins and carbohydrates, you will experience weight loss if you cut down on them. You will also reduce your risk of cancer, heart disease, diabetes, gallbladder problems, hypertension, and liver disease.

If you have a high blood cholesterol level, you have a greater chance of having a heart attack. Other factors can also increase your risk of heart attack—high blood pressure and cigarette smoking, for example—but high blood cholesterol is clearly a major dietary risk indicator.

Populations like ours with diets high in saturated fats and cholesterol tend to have high blood cholesterol levels. Individuals within these populations usually have greater risks of having heart attacks than people eating low-fat, low-cholesterol diets.

Eating extra saturated fat and cholesterol will increase blood cholesterol levels in most people. However, this will vary in different people according to genetic factors and the way in which each person's body uses cholesterol. Some people can consume diets high in saturated fats and cholesterol and still keep normal blood cholesterol levels. Other people are less fortunate, and have high blood cholesterol levels even if they eat low-fat, low-cholesterol diets.

There is controversy about what kind of diet will promote healthy Americans. But for the United States population as a whole, reduction in our current intake of total fat, saturated fat, and cholesterol is sensible. This suggestion is especially appropriate for people who have high blood pressure or who smoke. (See Appendix A for the fat and cholesterol content of different foods.)

Even though cholesterol itself is not a fat, cholesterol levels in the body are greatly affected by fat; cholesterol is, therefore, often associated with fat in food.

HOW TO REDUCE THE DANGERS OF FATS AND OILS

There are a number of ways that you can reduce the dangers associated with certain types of fats and oils. Some of these include maintaining a diet low in fat and cholesterol, exercising, supplementing your diet with niacin and lecithin, and testing your blood for fat and cholesterol.

The American Heart Association's booklet *Grocery Guide* offers tips about how to evaluate food and beverage labels in terms of fat and cholesterol. I spoke with a number of nutritionists who felt that some ingredients do not support healthy eating habits even though they may not increase your risk for cardiovascular disease. These ingredients have been italicized.

Acceptable Ingredients:

- Carob powder.
- Cocoa.
- Corn oil.
- *Cottonseed oil.*
- *Diglycerides.*
- Hydrolyzed ingredients.
- *Monoglycerides.*
- Nonfat dry milk or solids.

- Safflower oil.
- Sesame oil.
- Skim milk.
- Soybean oil (*partially hydrogenated*).
- Sunflower oil.

Unacceptable Ingredients:

- Animal fat.
- Butter.
- Cocoa butter.
- Coconut oil.
- Cream.
- Egg and egg-yolk solids.
- Hydrogenated fats and oils.
- Lard.
- Palm oil.
- Shortening.
- Whole-milk solids.

Drink Skim Milk

Research conducted at Pennsylvania State University indicates that skim milk may help to lower blood cholesterol. In a completed but unpublished study, a group of researchers including Arun Kilara, Ph.D., an associate professor of food science, "evaluated 82 volunteers, ages 30 to 75. Sixty-seven of the volunteers drank a quart of skim milk a day for eight weeks, and the rest formed a control group. One-third of the 67 people who drank skim milk showed a 7 to 8% drop in blood cholesterol." Some researchers believe that orotic acid, along with another unnamed component found in skim milk, inhibits your body's ability to produce cholesterol.

It is now known that palm and coconut oils (generally produced in Malaysia and Indonesia) may pose an even greater danger to cardiovascular health than animal fat. Palm kernel oil contains more than twice the level of saturated fat found in lard. Don't assume that all fats derived from non-animal sources are necessarily healthier for you. Many cooks like to use hardened fats since harder fats will reach higher temperatures when heated. Food will be cooked in a shorter period of time if you use hardened fats, resulting in a food that has absorbed less oil. As a result, the food will be crispier and less soggy.

Most medical doctors and mainstream researchers feel that atherosclerosis is irreversible and that high cholesterol levels can be reduced only through a change of diet or through drug therapy. (Cholestyramine and cholestipol are two of the most commonly prescribed drugs for high cholesterol according to *Time* magazine.)

There are a growing number of physicians, particularly those who practice what is commonly known as orthomolecular medicine, a term coined by Linus Pauling, who believe that abnormal levels of "bad" LDL (low-density lipoprotein) cholesterol result from a deficiency in certain vitamins and minerals that are essential to metabolizing and utilizing cholesterol properly.

Modify Your Diet

There are a number of ways to reduce your cholesterol levels effectively. You can start by keeping your daily cholesterol intake to 100 milligrams for each 1,000 calories you consume. No more than 300 milligrams of cholesterol should be consumed each day. You should avoid the following foods, which are high in cholesterol: eggs, organ meats such as kidneys and liver, shrimp, squid, lobster, mackerel, blue crab, and salmon. Clams, mussels, and shrimp are generally classified with those foods that are very high in cholesterol, yet are comparatively lower than most others in that group. Whereas an average hamburger can contain as much as 140 milligrams of cholesterol, an equal amount of clams (about

3½ ounces) will contain 40 to 60 milligrams of cholesterol. The same amount of mussels will contain from 60 to 90 milligrams of cholesterol, while 3½ ounces of shrimp will have about 90 milligrams of cholesterol.

Try to avoid making poor food choices. Get the facts before choosing a particular product. For example, you should avoid using highly saturated vegetable oils like palm and coconut oils. Instead, use monounsaturated fats (found in olive oil) and polyunsaturated fats (found in soybean and corn oil) since these seem to reduce blood cholesterol levels. Without getting proper information, many people replace high cholesterol foods like meat either with other high cholesterol foods like veal or with foods that are high in salt and fat like hard cheese. I would recommend using skim milk and low-fat milk products instead of whole milk.

Other foods such as oat bran have been shown to lower cholesterol levels. Pectin, a substance found in many fruits and vegetables, has been shown to reduce cholesterol in the blood effectively. Pectin has been found to reduce cholesterol even more effectively than wheat bran. Eat foods high in pectin, such as apples and blueberries, or use 1½ ounces of pectin daily. This is available in health food stores. Finally, you may wish to take certain nutritional supplements. Citing clinical evidence, researchers and physicians have claimed that high doses of vitamins B_3 and C can lower cholesterol levels, as can mineral supplements containing calcium, zinc, chronium, and selenium.

Exercise

Regular exercise is important for good health. Exercising will increase HDLs (the good cholesterol) and will lower triglyceride levels in your blood by utilizing any excess that you have for energy. You will experience many health benefits not only by exercising, but also by going on a diet that is low in cholesterol and fat. If you cannot go on a low-fat diet, at least try to reduce your fat intake. Refer to Appendix A for the fat and cholesterol content of different foods.

Take Supplements

How will supplementing your diet with niacin, lecithin, vitamin C, and vitamin B_6 help to reduce the dangers of fats? Having extremely high cholesterol levels seems to warrant the use of niacin. Over the last thirty years niacin has been shown to be helpful in treating high cholesterol problems. The best way to increase your niacin intake is to increase your intake of foods high in niacin such as natural peanut butter, potatoes, squash, whole grains, and legumes. When used in very high doses, this vitamin (B_3) usually takes the form known as nicotinic acid. The greatest benefits can be achieved when niacin supplementation is used in combination with a well-balanced diet, proper exercise, and a healthy mental attitude and lifestyle. High doses of niacin can have various side effects, so it should be used under the guidance of a nutritionist or a nutrition-oriented physician. While niacin is very effective in lowering blood cholesterol, it also increases the levels of uric acid and glucose in the blood and can even cause liver damage. The increase in uric acid levels can lead to gout, a form of arthritis.

In addition to supplementing your diet with niacin, you may wish to include vitamin C in your program. Studies conducted at Tufts University's Human Nutrition Research Center On Aging support the concept that increasing your intake of vitamin C may positively affect the heart and circulation. The study examined the effects of supplements and food intake on 680 men and women over sixty years of age. The researchers found that HDL cholesterol, the kind that is beneficial to your circulatory system, began to rise when more than 120 milligrams of vitamin C were taken each day. Those who used more than 1,000 milligrams of vitamin C each day had an average increase of 8 percent in the amount of HDL in their blood when compared with those individuals consuming under 120 milligrams. Vitamin B_6, along with EPA and DHA (unsaturated omega-3 fatty acids), is also important in reducing the negative effects of a high-fat diet.

Test for Blood Fat Levels

There is an old saying that ignorance of the truth is a poor excuse. Keeping this in mind, it is a good idea to find out whether your blood levels of fats and fat-related substances are within a safe range. The National Cholesterol Education Program, under the auspices of the National Heart, Lung, and Blood Institute, has begun a program to educate both the public and physicians on the importance of having blood tests after age twenty to determine cholesterol levels. The tests should not only measure total cholesterol levels, but also indicate HDL and LDL levels. Once you know about your cholesterol and blood pressure, you will have the necessary information to modify your dietary habits and lifestyle. Healthy women should not only have a baseline cholesterol test by age twenty, but should *continue* to have a test at least once every five years until they are forty. After age forty, they should have their cholesterol checked every three years. If you have a history of heart disease in your family, you may wish to discuss more frequent cholesterol checks with your physician.

What should your total cholesterol count be? Remember that cholesterol is measured in milligrams per deciliter (mg/dl). According to the National Cholesterol Education Program, a cholesterol level that is under 200 mg/dl indicates that you are probably eating properly and that you should repeat this blood test every five years. If your cholesterol level is 200–239 mg/dl, then you are moving into a borderline risk category for coronary heart disease (CHD); however, if your cholesterol level is 240 mg/dl or more, then you are moving into a high risk area.

The healthiest cholesterol levels for children are not as clear. Most physicians agree that a cholesterol level of 176 milligrams per deciliter of blood serum is high for children; however, there is no consensus on which cholesterol levels would be considered normal for children. Many public health experts feel that 140 to 150 milligrams would generally be a desirable level in children. For years many physicians believed that children would naturally outgrow high cholesterol levels; however, mounting evidence now shows that cholesterol levels in childhood may be the best indicator of high cholesterol levels and heart disease in adults.

You may recall that the lower your levels of high-density lipoproteins (HDL), the greater your risk for heart disease. It is important that your HDL levels be at least 35 mg/dl or higher. Even if you have a high total cholesterol level, having higher HDL levels allows you more flexibility in your diet.

Whereas having higher levels of HDLs is beneficial, the opposite is true of low-density lipoproteins (LDLs). Your LDL levels should be under 130 mg/dl. When these levels range from 130 mg/dl to 159 mg/dl, you are a borderline risk. When your LDL levels reach 160 mg/dl or above, you are at high risk for heart disease. If your LDL levels are in the high risk range, it is important to have these levels checked regularly. It is also advisable to go on a low-fat diet.

In addition to finding out your total cholesterol count and your HDL and LDL levels, you should also be aware of your triglyceride levels. Although the connection between diet and triglyceride levels has not been as clearly established as that between diet and blood cholesterol levels, it is best to keep triglyceride levels within a safe range. Having triglyceride levels of 250 mg/dl or above is a sign that something is off balance. These test results may indicate problems such as hypertension, hypoglycemia, excessive weight, or low HDL levels.

Unfortunately, making a proper diagnosis from your blood test is not always easy. A physician's uncertainty when interpreting your blood tests, together with imprecision in some lab results, has impeded efforts to reduce the incidence of high cholesterol. A survey conducted in 1986 by the National Heart, Lung, and Blood Institute found that as many as 50 to 75 percent of physicians failed to suggest dietary changes or to provide drug treatment for patients with dangerously high cholesterol levels. It is apparent that even with new information arriving on the scene, many physicians are confused about what a dangerously high level of cholesterol is. According to an October 1987 article in *Time* magazine, "measurements of cholesterol levels can be off as much as 300% depending on the test, the lab and even what the patient had to eat and drink in the previous twelve hours." In addition to this confusion, many clients who were told that they were in a safe to borderline high risk range may actually be at higher risk than the test initially indicated. This is due to the fact that some people may smoke or have a history of heart disease in their family. Males are also at a higher risk than females.

DANGERS ASSOCIATED WITH HEAT AND OXIDATION

In addition to being concerned about the amount of fat in your diet, you should also be careful about heating oils to high temperatures and about exposing them to oxygen. The way in which oils are manufactured, processed, and used affects their safety and nutritional value.

The Formation of Trans-Fatty Acids

Remember that you should avoid heating fats and oils to very high temperatures since certain unwanted reactions may take place and certain unwanted end products may result. When fats or oils are heated to high temperatures, a slight change in the molecular structure of the fat molecule takes place. This change results in the formation of an unnatural fatty acid known as a trans-fatty acid. The prefix "trans" describes the changed molecular configuration compared with the normal or "cis" configuration. This new molecular structure can change the properties and functions of the fat.

Because the "trans" configuration is more stable than the "cis" configuration, your body cannot easily convert it to other fats that are needed. Even though the "trans" form takes up the same space as the "cis" form, it doesn't perform any of the functions of the cis-fatty acids and actually blocks the cis-essential fatty acids. As a result, certain important functions requiring cis-fatty acids cannot be properly completed. For example, energy and electron exchange reactions cannot take place. Whereas cis-fatty acids can be used either for important parts of the cell membrane or as fuel, trans-fatty acids are useful only as fuel.

Trans-fatty acids pose a particular danger because they are broken down in your body by enzymes at a much slower rate than cis-fatty acids. Why is this dangerous? When trans-fatty acids rise to high levels in your body, they interfere with the essential functions that cis-fatty acids usually perform. Organs such as the heart may not be able to function adequately. If you were to experience a crisis or great stress, the decreased functioning ability of your heart or of another organ might prove fatal.

Trans-fatty acids may damage the protective barrier around the cell and thus increase the permeability of the cell membranes. Certain molecules that should remain in the cell might now be able to escape, while other undesirable molecules that previously were not permitted to enter the cell can now do so.

In addition to posing a threat to the cell membranes, trans-fatty acids may aggravate an essential fatty acid deficiency that already exists by inhibiting various enzyme processes that are essential to good health, particularly the transformation of fatty acids into other essential molecules. This may ultimately have a negative effect on the production of prostaglandins, which will affect blood pressure, platelet stickiness, and blood clotting.

It is easy to see why the formation of trans-fatty acids under high temperatures is detrimental to your health. These substances are fat molecules that have been altered to a form not normally found in nature. They are the wrong size, shape, and configuration to perform the functions for which fats are necessary.

Diseases Associated With Trans-Fatty Acids

A correlation between consumption of trans-fatty acids and atherosclerosis has been documented. Trans-fatty acids can increase blood triglyceride and cholesterol levels. High levels of triglycerides have been shown to play a role in the development of cardiovascular disease. In addition, many forms of cancer have been associated with high-fat diets. Statistics indicate that the incidence of cancer has increased with our consumption of hydrogenated vegetable oils, which form trans-fatty acids when heated. After viewing the available evidence, some researchers have concluded that some cancers involve a functional deficiency of the essential fatty acids. It is possible that this functional deficiency is somehow related to high levels of trans-fatty acids.

Fortunately, the body has ways of breaking down many of the trans-fatty acids and minimizing their damage. Nevertheless, they are extremely undesirable. I would advise you to avoid using fried and partially hydrogenated oils, which can make trans-fatty acids.

The Formation of Free Radicals

Free radicals is the name given to certain chemically reactive molecules that your body must deal with every day. To be specific, a free radical is an element or molecule with an unpaired electron. Research on fats and oils has enabled us to understand more clearly the role that free radicals play in health and disease. Free radicals must be controlled in the body; if they are not limited and localized, they can cause chain reactions that may create abnormal toxic products in your body and cause faulty biochemical functions and various diseases. Not all free radicals are dangerous—some play a role in various normal metabolic reactions. Free radicals serve as intermediaries in the thousands of chemical reactions that take place in your body every day. By using these free radicals in its chemical reactions, your body prevents them from causing damage in other areas.

There are a number of substances created by your body to keep these free radicals in check, and other substances that your body can use to scavenge free radicals. Two enzymes that help to control free radicals are glutathione peroxidase and superoxide dismutase (SOD). Other enzymes, as well as vitamins C and E, will scavenge for free radicals. These free radical scavengers are used by the body to neutralize the free radicals and to prevent them from causing damage.

The Dangers Associated With Free Radicals

When a fat or oil has been manufactured or stored improperly, a process known as oxidation takes place. A rancid taste indicates that the oil has been oxidized. When a fat has been oxidized and broken down, a peroxide forms. Free radicals are commonly found in fats that have been peroxidized such as those often found in atherosclerotic plaques. A few of the health problems associated with free radical damage are:

- Premature aging.

- Age pigment accumulation that can "choke off" brain cells and cause brown age spots to form on your skin.

- Alteration of the structure of proteins, fats, DNA, and RNA. DNA and RNA are the nucleic acids responsible for your genetic blueprint.

- Cancer. This results from the mutations in your DNA due to free radical activity.

- Abnormal blood clotting. This results from the destruction of certain anti-clotting hormones by free radicals.

- Cross-linking, which can make your tissues brittle and stiff. This, in turn, can lead to cerebral hemorrhage, general loss of flexibility, and emphysema.

- Arthritis. This results from the damage done by hydroxyl radicals, the most powerful of all oxidants.

Preventing Free Radical Damage

To prevent free radical damage, it is important that you reduce your caloric intake. If you eat foods containing fewer calories, your body will produce fewer free radicals in metabolism. One of the best ways to do this is to reduce your intake of fats and oils. A healthy, well-balanced diet will enable your body to keep free radicals under control.

Studies have shown, however, that Japanese fishermen and Eskimos living a traditional lifestyle may have high levels of highly unsaturated fatty acids in their tissues and still have a low incidence of the degenerative diseases generally associated with free radical damage. So eat well, avoid highly refined and processed foods, and make sure that any fats and oils that you use have been properly stored. Taking nutritional supplements can help you prevent or at least reduce the effect of free radicals on your body. Nutrients that use or tie up free radicals are generally called antioxidants and include:

- Vitamins A, C, E, B_1, B_5, and B_6.

- The amino acids cysteine and tyrosine.

- Pycnogenol. This pine bark extract is patented and available in many natural food stores. According to its manufacturer, it is unique in that it penetrates the blood-brain barrier, acts within minutes, and remains in the bloodstream for seventy-two hours. It is the only oxygenated radical scavenger.

- Catechols, which are found in potatoes and bananas.

- Phenolics (compounds chemically similar to BHT), which are found in grapes and other fruit.

- The minerals zinc and selenium.

Hydrogenation

One of the ways that commercial food processors damage the nutritional value of the essential fatty acids is through a process called **hydrogenation**. Hydrogenation is a process in which an oil is artificially hardened. In the presence of a metal catalyst, the oil reacts with hydrogen gas under pressure after six to eight hours at very high temperatures. The most commonly used catalyst in this process is nickel, but copper or platinum may be used as well.

Total hydrogenation of an oil results in a substance that has no essential fatty acid activity, does not spoil, and can be heated, fried, cooked, roasted, or baked. Hydrogenation allows food processors to use cheaper oil and give it any desired texture—semi-liquid or solid, spreadable or firm. Margarines, though used essentially as "imitation butter," often will have a slight rancid taste, especially in the summer. Although butter may also have this rancid taste, it will disappear when the butter is heated by evaporating the part of the butter that gives it this disagreeable taste. Heating margarine will not have this same effect since its rancidity comes from a different source. Some researchers feel that fully hydrogenated fat may be useful even for natural foods enthusiasts, since it does not go rancid and is free of the trans-fatty acids that pose a health risk in other types of fats.

The Dangers of Hydrogenation

Although hydrogenated fats do have some unique uses, you should not consider using them. Hydrogenated fats contain altered molecules created from fatty acids and also contain fatty acid fragments as a result of the hydrogenation process. Some of these altered fatty acids and molecules may be toxic, and there is always the possibility that the fat may have been contaminated by some of the metal catalyst. It is best to avoid using products made from hydrogenated fats whenever possible, especially since there are products containing high quality oil available.

Hydrogenated fats and oils have many commercial uses. They can be fried over and over and can be stored for long periods of time. If you look at the list of ingredients on any candy wrapper, hydrogenated fat is generally the primary ingredient. The reason for the widespread use of hydrogenated fat is that it acts as a hardening agent and prevents melting in products like chocolate (except in very warm weather), while it enables the product to "melt in your mouth, not in your hands." Hydrogenated fats are also used in food processing; the oil is heated so that oil-soluble factors can be extracted from onion, garlic, and other plants.

Partial Hydrogenation

Some food processors use fats that have been only partially hydrogenated. Both researchers and nutritionists are concerned about the safety of these products. When fats are partially hydrogenated, a large number of compounds are produced, few of which have been studied. It is not known what effects, if any, these compounds have on your health. It is literally impossible to control the production of chemicals during the hydrogenation process, and it's impossible to predict how much of a particular compound will be produced in any one batch of partially hydrogenated fat. Among the most undesirable of the products resulting from the partial hydrogenation process are trans-fatty acids. Remember that these fatty acids can negatively affect numerous essential processes in the body. Although partially hydrogenated oils are used in many processed foods, you will probably recall that this process is used to make shortenings, shortening oils, and margarines.

Many consumer advocates and authorities on fats and oils feel that if partial hydrogenation were introduced as a new process today, it would not be approved by the Food and Drug Administration. This process, however, has been in use since the 1930s. Besides having a long tradition, partial hydrogenation has the support of a powerful lobby in the food processing and oil industry.

Fried Foods

Frying (actually deep-frying) involves cooking over dry heat. When you boil food in water, it will moisten the food; however, when you fry food in fat, it coats the food rather than penetrating it. The oil used in frying is actually a medium for transferring heat to the food. Frying, if done properly, may not make food greasy and will not be a health hazard. Unfortunately, food is seldom fried properly, and that is why problems arise.

Dangers Associated With Fried Foods

The primary problem with frying stems from the rapid changes that take place when unsaturated fats are exposed to light, heat, and air. Unlike unsaturated fats, saturated fats remain stable in spite of environmental changes. So even though unsaturated fats are generally healthier than saturated fats, it is the saturated fats that are more desirable for frying. It is best to avoid any liquid oils when frying since these are high in unsaturated fats. When unsaturated fats are heated to high temperatures, there are a number of toxic substances that are produced in addition to the trans-fatty acids. It is not easy to identify many of these toxic substances, and some of them remain a mystery. Of all the ways in which we use fats, probably none is as widespread nor produces as many toxic substances as frying in oil. Whether oil is fried in open air or in an air-free environment, it will produce foreign substances—none of which are desirable. In commercial uses of frying, the oil is reused again and again regardless of whether it is saturated or unsaturated. Reusing oil is highly inadvisable since it results in the formation of many altered substances—some of them toxic.

If you fry foods often, you should not repeatedly use the same oil. It is not difficult to tell whether an oil has been overused, overheated, or abused in cooking. Such oil will become dark in color, and food that has been fried in it will have a strong odor and flavor. Any oil in this state should not be used. It is best to fry only occasionally and, when you do, to use a saturated fat such as butter, coconut oil, or palm kernel oil.

Some people mistakenly believe that frying causes oil to become more saturated. Saturates may occur naturally in fats and oils or as a result of hydrogenation, but no matter what negative effects frying does have, it alone *cannot* increase saturation.

Reducing the Dangers of Frying

If you are willing to experiment, you can learn to fry in a way that makes the food safe and tasty. As you may know, much of the food that you eat in Chinese restaurants is prepared in a metal pan called a wok. The shape of the wok is designed to spread heat evenly and intensely without burning. In traditional Chinese cooking, the first thing that is put into the wok is water, not oil. Chinese cooks use water first before adding oil for two reasons: it keeps the temperature down and forms steam that protects the oil from air, reducing oxidation. It is the oxidation that makes the American method of frying unhealthy. In European cooking, vegetables are placed in a frying pan before the oil is added as a means of protecting the oil from oxidation and overheating. Since Chinese and European cooking require that you stir the food while it's in the pan, more care is required for its preparation than for food cooked by deep-frying. The benefits of cooking in the Chinese or European manner, however, are great; your food will be healthier, retain more of its natural flavors, and have less of the burnt taste so often associated with fried food.

CONCLUSION

In 1988 the most comprehensive report on the relationship between diet and health ever compiled by the federal government was published. Surgeon General Everett C. Koop called on Americans to reduce their consumption of fat and increase their consumption of fiber by using whole grains, fruits, and vegetables in place of animal proteins. The 712-page Surgeon General's Report on Nutrition and Health, released in July, concluded that diet was associated with the cause of death of at least two-thirds of the 2.1 million Americans who died in 1987 (a total of over 1.4 million people).

Never before has an official government document been as explicit in attacking the role of animal products in the human diet. The literature supporting the recommendation that Americans reduce their fat and cholesterol intake clearly indicates that "the major dietary sources of fat in the American diet are meat, poultry, fish, dairy products, and fats and oils. . . . Dietary cholesterol is found only in foods of animal origin, such as eggs, meat, poultry, fish, and dairy products."

It is clear from the most up-to-date research, and from the recommendations of nutritionists and doctors, that you will benefit most if you pay attention to the amount and quality of the fats and oils you use. If you use this book as a reference text on a regular basis and follow its recommendations, you will have the tools for reducing your risk of cancer, cardiovascular disease, stroke, heart attack, and many other diseases. Fats and oils are essential to life, and if used properly and effectively, they can help you heal and build and maintain a healthy lifestyle. Keeping this in mind, you should choose oils that are high in essential fatty acids and store them appropriately. Use the next chapter as a guide to choosing oils that will enhance the nutritional value and flavor of your meal when stored and used correctly.

6
Getting to Know Your Fats and Oils

When you shop in a supermarket or health food store, there are many brands and types of oils to choose from. There is canola oil, coconut oil, corn oil, cottonseed oil, flaxseed oil, mustard oil, peanut oil, safflower oil, sesame oil, soybean oil, sunflower oil, and wheat germ oil—to name a few! Because each variety has its own unique properties and gives food a distinct flavor, you can use them for different purposes. Some oils are better for frying, some for sautéing, and others for baking. Some oils have a longer shelf life than others. You will be able to make a better choice if you are aware of the positive and negative effects that each oil may have.

CANOLA (RAPESEED) OIL

At one time this oil contained high levels of erucic acid, which has been found to cause fatty degeneration of the adrenal glands, heart, kidneys, and thyroid. In recent years new varieties of the seed have been developed that are much lower in erucic acid; even so, this oil is not your best choice since any amount of erucic acid that is used in food preparation is too much.

COCONUT OIL

This is among the most saturated of all the vegetable oils (91 percent saturated), while it is comprised of only 3 percent linoleic acid. Comparing the saturation of coconut oil with lard will give you an idea of how saturated it really is. Whereas saturated acids comprise 39 to 40 percent of lard, twice this amount makes up coconut oil. Because of its high level of saturation, coconut oil is solid at room temperature and remains stable in frying and storage. Since coconut oil will melt only within a small range of temperatures, it will change from solid to liquid and back without becoming soft between the two consistencies. This adds a brittle quality to the confections that it is used in. Coconut oil comes from the nut of the coconut palm, which grows wild in the Pacific Islands—especially in Malaysia, the Philippines, and Indonesia. The palm also grows on the southwest coast of North America. The fifty to seventy-five coconuts that each palm produces annually are first cracked and then dried. After this is done, the remaining pulp of the coconut, called copra, is 65 to 70 percent fat. Copra will be of the best quality if it is dried in hot-air dryers, in the sun, or over fires. The oil is extracted by expeller pressing the copra or by solvent extraction. Although it is used in some food products, coconut oil is used primarily in cosmetics and confections, and as an oil in Swedish massage.

CORN OIL

Corn oil is one of the most popular of the oils and has been used commercially in the United States for many years. You may remember the television commercials that used to tout how high corn oil was in polyunsaturates (85 percent unsaturated). Its high polyunsaturate level made this oil the natural choice for making margarine. Although corn oil contains less linoleic acid than other oils, it is still high at 56 percent. Natural corn oil has a rich, buttery flavor and aroma that may limit its use in foods that call for a more neutral flavor.

Natural corn oil may begin to foam in deep-frying, so it is not the best choice for this type of cooking either. Since heavily processed corn oil has had much of its natural flavor and aroma removed, these limitations, of course, do not apply; however, processed corn oil is a nutritionally inferior product.

Most of the corn oil that you use—even the natural variety—is a product of those industries that use corn for more profitable items, such as cereal production, and for its starch (used in glucose manufacturing). Most corn oil is extracted from the germ of the corn kernel and is called corn germ oil, while some is extracted from the whole kernel, which contains oil under the hull, and is called corn gluten oil. Corn gluten oil is dark red and has a strong, almost popcorny aroma, while corn germ oil is light yellow and has a lighter, cornier flavor. Unlike some other oils, corn oil is very stable even though it has a high content of unsaturated fats and linoleic acid. Corn oil gets its stability primarily from its high vitamin E content, which prevents oxidation. It's a rich oil that is a favorite choice for baking breads and pie crusts, dressing salads, and sautéing.

COTTONSEED OIL

Even though cottonseed oil is found in many processed foods, including potato chips and other snacks, it is among the most undesirable of the oils. Cottonseed oil contains cyclopropene fatty acid—a potentially toxic component. This fatty acid slows down sexual maturity and can cause female reproductive functions to stop when found in higher quantities. It may have harmful effects upon the gallbladder and liver. This fatty acid also destroys enzymes essential to the functioning of highly unsaturated fatty acids. Cyclopropene fatty acid is especially dangerous when used in the processing of peanut products, as when peanuts are roasted in cottonseed oil. Peanuts may contain fungus-produced chemicals called aflatoxins, which are known to cause cancer; unfortunately, cyclopropene fatty acid can greatly enhance their carcinogenic power.

In addition to cyclopropene fatty acid, pesticides may be a worry for those who use cottonseed oil. One of the problems with modern farming techniques is the level of pesticide residues found on many fruits, vegetables, and grains. Of all the foods that have been sprayed with pesticides, the pesticide residues found in cottonseed oil are the highest. This is a result of the intensive overspraying by cotton farmers to control boll weevils and other cotton pests.

Cottonseed oil is also an unpopular choice because it contains gossypol. This complex component of cottonseed oil may induce shortness of breath, irritation of the digestive tract, and retention of water in the lungs, and, when taken in high levels, may even cause paralysis in extreme cases.

FLAXSEED OIL

This really is the finest of the oils. Unfortunately, due to its very high levels of essential fatty acids, flaxseed oil is very unstable and spoils easily. Use flaxseed oil only in recipes that do not use heat. It can be used topically as a healing agent and as a prevention against cardiovascular disease by helping to reduce cholesterol levels. If you use flax oil, it is important that you store it properly.

Using flaxseed oil can be beneficial to you in a number of ways. It is nature's richest and "cleanest" source of omega-3 fatty acids. The benefits of omega-3 fatty acids were discussed in Chapter 4. Flaxseed oil may help reduce health problems by greatly lowering the level of triglycerides in your blood and slightly lowering your cholesterol levels.

MUSTARD OIL

Avoid using mustard oil on food since it has a high erucic acid content. Refer to the section on canola oil for further information on this problem.

PEANUT OIL

Next to safflower oil, peanut oil is probably the most commonly used oil in commercial food processing. Peanut oil is a by-product of the peanut industry, which uses the "expeller press" or "solvent extract" method to extract the oil from the less useful nuts. Peanut oil is among the highest of the oils in saturated fat (20 percent), and is made up of only about 30 percent linoleic acid. This combination makes peanut oil among the most stable. Expeller-pressed peanut oil has a longer shelf life than expeller-pressed safflower oil, although the reverse is true when safflower oil is in its refined form.

Some prelimary studies, especially one reported in November 1976 in "Chemical and Engineering News," indicate that peanut oil, though an unsaturated fat, may contribute to atherosclerosis. These, of course, were preliminary studies; however, if you cook with oil, you might want to choose another variety.

SAFFLOWER OIL

This oil is the most popular vegetable oil in the natural foods industry, although it is only in recent years that it has become better known in the regular market place. Because the safflower plant belongs to the sunflower family, their oils are very similar. Safflower oil is probably the lightest and least flavorful of the oils, though it does have a pleasant, slightly nutty taste. Many people who have just been introduced to expeller-pressed oils and natural foods will choose this oil because it is most similar to the highly processed oils in color, flavor, and odor.

Safflower oil is 94 percent unsaturated, perhaps the highest of all the oils. Its linoleic acid content is 78 percent, making it the highest of all oils in this area as well. As good as this may sound, there is also a drawback. Remember that unsaturated fats tend to spoil faster than saturated fats. An oil as highly unsaturated as safflower will therefore have a shorter shelf life than other oils. Because it is the least expensive of the oils, most natural food processors and packaged food manufacturers use safflower oil in their products. Safflower oil is best refrigerated in the summer months to prevent rancidity, and similarly should be kept in a very cool place in the winter.

A light oil, safflower oil is suitable for sautéing and for making mayonnaise. It is not recommended for deep-frying since its flavor does not remain stable under high temperatures.

SESAME OIL

As mentioned in Chapter 1, sesame oil is one of the oldest oils produced. Not only was this oil used by the Chinese as a food, but it was also essential to the production of ink and cosmetics. Sesame oil is generally available in a dark or light form. The dark variety is prepared from seeds that have been roasted before pressing. You might recognize the toasted, smoky flavor of this oil in an entree prepared by a Chinese restaurant. It is this type of sesame oil that is most commonly used in Chinese cooking. The lighter variety has a milder, nutty flavor and can be used in a variety of ways. Although sesame oil is one of the poorest sources of linoleic acid (42 percent) among the oils, it is 87 percent unsaturated. This and other factors make it very stable and highly resistant to oxidation.

Very little sesame oil is manufactured in the United States. Most of the seeds are imported from Central America and pressed in small quantities. Importation has grown in recent years with the increased interest in Japanese, Vietnamese, and Korean cuisine. With the exception of certain types of olive oil, sesame oil is the most expensive of the oils. It is a light oil that is generally used for deep-frying, for sautéing grains, noodles, and vegetables, and for salad dressings.

SOYBEAN OIL

Until the late 1970s, most people had thought of soybeans only as something to feed cattle or as something used to make soy sauce. Until World War II, soybean oil was virtually unknown even among commercial food processors. In little more than forty years, this oil has become the source of over 65 percent of all oil used commercially. Originally the United States had imported most of its soybean oil from China and Indonesia; however, during the war the United States increased its production of soybean oil and is now the largest exporter of this oil in the world. Soybeans are not a popular choice for expeller pressing, since the oil content of soybeans is only 16 to 18 percent. For this reason, chemical extraction is the most common means of obtaining this oil in commercial production. While commercially extracted soybean oil is a clear light color, the expeller-pressed variety is a dark yellow with a light green tinge. It gets its green tone from its chlorophyll content. Soybean oil is 50 percent linoleic acid, and is highly susceptible to oxidation. Of all the oils, soy oil has the strongest flavor. You would not want to use the unrefined variety since its taste does not remain stable. Some have even likened its taste to paint or fish. Commercially, the refined variety is most commonly used in processed foods, and is either hydrogenated or partially hydrogenated. Natural food shoppers will seldom use it in frying, since the food must be eaten immediately or it will develop disagreeable flavors and odors. This oil is best used in salad dressings or for baking where the taste is not as strong.

SUNFLOWER OIL

Most oil-producing seeds cannot be produced in cold climates, but sunflower oil is one of the exceptions. This oil is generally produced in Canada and is of great commercial importance in the Soviet Union. Although it is not among the most popular oils available in the United States, natural foods enthusiasts often choose it for salads or for frying. The composition of sunflower oil will vary with each purchase since many varieties of this plant are used in the production of sunflower oil. Sunflower oil and safflower oil are quite similar, with the former having a little stronger flavor. Like safflower oil, sunflower oil is highly unsaturated—92 percent—and is 72 percent linoleic acid. Sunflower oil stores better than safflower oil since it is more resistant to oxidation. Sunflower and corn oil are the only oils that are indigenous to North America.

WHEAT GERM OIL

In the early part of the twentieth century when the "health food" movement was in its formative stages, wheat germ oil was often touted as a valuable nutritional supplement. Recent research has shown that this praise was not misdirected. Studies originally conducted from 1949 to 1969 by Thomas Cureton, Ph.D., professor and director of the Physical Fitness Institute at the University of Illinois, found that a substance in wheat germ oil called octacosanol helped to improve endurance and speed reaction time, provided glycogen to help strengthen muscles, and reduced oxygen debt. Other preliminary studies have shown that octacosanol may lower cholesterol, aid in the treatment of certain neurological disorders, increase fertility, prevent spontaneous abortion, and relieve toxemia brought on by pregnancy.

Although minute amounts of this element can now be obtained from other plant sources, octacosanol supplements were originally derived from wheat germ. Much of the octacosanol available in health food stores is derived from other plant sources, but manufacturers are reluctant to name what they are. Natural octacosanol does not appear anywhere in nature other than in unprocessed wheat germ oil; however, your body can derive octacosanol from certain other elements found in plants. Octacosanol, a member of a family of waxy alcohols, has been shown through clinical studies to have great potential therapeutic value. Dr. Helmut Prahl, executive director for the Dynatron Research Foundation in Madison, Wisconsin, says that diseases of the central nervous system generally respond to octacosanol. Even conditions as diverse as arthritis, multiple sclerosis, amyotrophic lateral sclerosis, stroke, cerebral palsy, muscular dystrophy, and Parkinson's disease have shown symptomatic reductions with octacosanol supplementation.

Octacosanol is generally used in some synthesized form since it occurs in wheat germ in very low concentrations and is costly to isolate and extract on a commercial scale. Studies have shown that octacosanol is the substance in wheat germ oil that increases endurance, performance, basal metabolism, and so on—not the vitamin E and polyunsaturated linoleic acid that are also found in wheat germ oil.

Refer to Table 6.1 for a comparison of the fat content of selected fats and oils. The fats are listed from lowest to highest saturated fat content. When you are preparing your meals, you can refer to Table 6.2 for a particular oil's best uses.

Studies have shown that having higher levels of polyunsaturates does not necessarily mean that one oil will be more effective than another in lowering blood cholesterol levels. These studies do indicate that all highly polyunsaturated oils will help to lower blood cholesterol levels, so choose your oils wisely.

Other factors to take into consideration when shopping for the best oil besides its level of saturation are the steps that were taken by the manufacturer and packager to preserve the quality and freshness of the oil and the stability of the particular oil when exposed to heat, light, and air.

HOW DO OILS GO BAD?

Although fats are essential for good health, they can also be dangerous to your health if they are not stored properly. Both linoleic and linolenic acid are very unstable and can be destroyed easily by heat, light, and air. It is for this reason that knowledge and attention to detail are essential in the manufacturing, packaging, and storage of any oils high in the essential fatty acids. The nuts and seeds that most oils are derived from are incredibly efficient storage units. They provide an environment so stable that oils can remain fresh in them for years.

Table 6.1   The Fat Content of Fats and Oils

Product (1 Tablespoon)	Saturated Fatty Acids (Grams)	Cholesterol (Milligrams)	Polyunsaturated Fatty Acids (Grams)	Monounsaturated Fatty Acids (Grams)
Rapeseed oil (canola oil)	0.9	0	4.5	7.6
Safflower oil	1.2	0	10.1	1.6
Sunflower oil	1.4	0	5.5	6.2
Peanut butter, smooth	1.5	0	2.3	3.7
Corn oil	1.7	0	8.0	3.3
Olive oil	1.8	0	1.1	9.9
Sunflower oil, hydrogenated	1.8	0	4.9	6.3
Margarine, liquid, bottled	1.8	0	5.1	3.9
Margarine, soft, tub	1.8	0	3.9	4.8
Sesame oil	1.9	0	5.7	5.4
Soybean oil	2.0	0	7.9	3.2
Margarine, stick	2.1	0	3.6	5.1
Peanut oil	2.3	0	4.3	6.2
Cottonseed oil	3.5	0	7.1	2.4
Lard	5.0	12	1.4	5.8
Beef tallow	6.4	14	0.5	5.3
Palm oil	6.7	0	1.3	5.0
Butter	7.1	31	0.4	3.3
Cocoa butter	8.1	0	0.4	3.3
Palm kernel	11.1	0	0.2	1.5
Coconut oil	11.8	0	0.2	0.8

Sources: *Composition of Foods: Fats and Oils—Raw • Processed • Prepared, Agriculture Handbook 8-4.* United States Department of Agriculture, Science and Education Administration (June 1979).

   Composition of Foods: Legumes and Legume Products—Raw • Processed • Prepared, Agriculture Handbook 8-16. United States Department of Agriculture, Human Nutrition Information Service (December 1986).

Table 6.2   Uses of Oils

Oils	Cooking	Baking	Frying	Sautéing	Sauces	Salads
Almond, refined	✔			✔	✔	✔
Apricot Kernel, refined	✔			✔	✔	✔
Avocado, refined	✔			✔	✔	✔
Corn, refined	✔	✔				✔
Corn, unrefined	✔	✔				
Flaxseed	No-heat recipes only					
Grapeseed, refined	✔		✔	✔		✔
Olive, "extra-virgin"	✔			✔	✔	✔
Peanut, refined	✔	✔	✔	✔	✔	
Peanut, unrefined	✔			✔	✔	
Pumpkinseed	No-heat recipes only					
High-Oleic Safflower, refined (mono)	✔	✔	✔	✔		✔
High-Oleic Safflower, unrefined (mono)	✔	✔	✔			✔
Regular Safflower, refined (poly)	✔	✔		✔		✔
Regular Safflower, unrefined (poly)	✔	✔				✔

Table 6.2—*Continued*

Oils	Cooking	Baking	Frying	Sautéing	Sauces	Salads
Sesame, refined	✔	✔		✔	✔	✔
Sesame, unrefined	✔	✔		✔	✔	✔
Sesame, unrefined, toasted	✔		✔	✔	✔	
Sesame, unrefined, golden toasted	✔		✔	✔	✔	
Soybean, refined	✔	✔				✔
High-Oleic Sunflower, refined (mono)	✔	✔	✔	✔		✔
High-Oleic Sunflower, unrefined (mono)	✔	✔	✔			
Regular Sunflower, refined (poly)	✔	✔		✔		✔
Walnut, refined	✔	✔		✔		✔

Source: Spectrum Naturals. Reprinted with permission.

*Cooking is the general item for all recipes such as casseroles, loafs, soups, etc.

Note: Refined and unrefined varieties of an oil may be used differently due to the strong aroma and flavor of unrefined oils. Most unrefined oils have a distinct flavor that can limit or enhance their use according to individual tastes.

When an oil becomes rancid, it is usually the result of oxidation (prolonged exposure to air). Oxidation causes the formation of peroxides and other foul-smelling and poor-tasting elements. Rancid oil not only smells and tastes bad, but is also dangerous in that it deteriorates blood cells and speeds up the aging process. Some of the other toxic products that are formed when rancidity (oxidation) takes place in unsaturated fatty acids are:

- Hydroperoxide polymers.

- Hydroperoxyaldehydes, which are the most highly toxic of all substances resulting from oxidation.

- Peroxides and ozonides, which not only are toxic to lung tissues, but can also be fatal in high levels.

Once oil is extracted, the breakdown process takes place quickly and the oil may easily become rancid. Creating conditions that will keep the oil fresh after extraction is very difficult and costly.

There are three basic elements that can cause an oil to become rancid: light, heat, and oxygen. Light is the most destructive of all the factors that affect essential fatty acids. You already have read how mixing an oil with oxygen causes it to become rancid. Light speeds up this process by 1,000 times. Chain reactions will begin to take place in the presence of light because there are now free radicals (discussed in Chapter 5). Free radical formation will cause essential fatty acids in the oil to break down into various components, some toxic and some nontoxic. Aldehydes and ketones are among the substances that are formed.

Many of the steps used to process oil actually contribute to its breakdown. High temperatures should be avoided when processing oil. If you think about the high temperatures that we use to fry with oil or about the processes used to refine, hydrogenate, and deodorize oils, it is no wonder that the normal shape of the oil's molecules is changed or that the essential fatty acids are ultimately destroyed.

PRESERVING THE QUALITY AND FRESHNESS OF OILS

The way in which an oil is manufactured and processed will partly determine its freshness and shelf life. Manufacturers sometimes expeller press their oils and package them with nitrogen to preserve their freshness.

Expeller Pressing

Expeller-pressed oils contain various substances that prevent rancidity. These natural preservatives help to prevent the oil from reacting with oxygen. The most common natural preservatives include vitamin E, lecithin, and sesamol, which is found in unrefined sesame oil. Vitamin E is particularly popular because it not only protects oil from rancidity over a period of months, it also prevents oil from going rancid once it is in your body. This reduces some of the risks normally associated with oil rancidity such as certain types of anemia and premature aging.

Nitrogen Packaging

A few of the companies that package natural oil will replace the air in the space at the top of the bottle with nitrogen. This is an effective way of preventing the rancidity that normally occurs from oxidation. Nitrogen is an inert gas that makes up 80 percent of the air we breath. Once you open an oil that has been packed with nitrogen, it is important to refrigerate it or store it in a cool, dry place. Make sure that the bottle is closed tight.

HOW TO TELL IF YOUR OILS ARE FRESH

By smelling or tasting an oil, you can accurately tell how fresh it is. Heavily processed oil has a bland to neutral odor, while a fresh expeller-pressed oil has a full aroma of olives, sesame seeds, peanuts, soybeans, or sunflowers. Rancid oil also has a sharp, almost bitter taste. Of course, heavily processed oil will not exhibit this quality since most of the nutrients have been removed from it, and preservatives have been added.

Have you ever eaten fried food or sunflower seeds that had a somewhat sharp or bitter taste? What you were probably tasting was rancid oil! Since oils are very unstable, the presence of oxygen—even in the absence of great heat or light—will cause essential fatty acids to break down. Consider the fact that an oil will be of a better quality when it is exposed to the least amount of light, heat, and oxygen. It is best, therefore, to purchase oils that have been expeller pressed (cold pressed). These oils should be packaged in dark bottles that exclude oxygen, and should be stored away from direct sunlight.

STORAGE TIME FOR DIFFERENT OILS

To get the greatest benefits from oils, it is important that their nutritional content be intact, and that they not be spoiled. Try to purchase oil in small quantities and store them appropriately. Certain oils can be bought in larger quantities than others because they have a different spoilage time. The spoilage time will vary because of the differences in the three unsaturated fatty acids. The most unstable and reactive of the unsaturated fatty acids is linolenic acid, followed by linoleic acid. The least reactive is the monounsaturated arachidonic acid. Flax oil is the most unstable of the commercial oils; it spoils the most rapidly due to its high linolenic acid content. Expeller-pressed oils will remain usable for four to six months (and perhaps longer) depending on how they are stored. Oils that have been heavily processed may keep for twice as long since they have fewer nutrients that can contribute to deterioration. These oils generally have BHT, BHA, propyl gallate, or other preservatives added to them.

How should you store particular types of oil? Since some oils will go bad quicker than other oils, you should be aware of their differences. Flax oil, for example, can be stored for three months in a cool, closed container. Once opened, this oil will keep for two to three weeks. Many people use sesame, sunflower, safflower, and pumpkin oils because they can be stored well for nine to twelve months in a cool, closed container. These oils will be good for two to three months after opening. Olive oil can be stored even longer—up to two years in a cool, closed container.

If you follow the guidelines provided in this chapter, you will be able to choose high quality oils, preserve their freshness through proper storage, and prepare meals with them in a way that creates fullness of flavor and optimal nutrition whether you are baking, frying, or sautéing.

7
Being a
Smart Consumer

As you might have guessed by now, eating whole natural foods does not guarantee that your diet is low in fats and oils. Even when avoiding heavily processed foods, you may be taking in large amounts of saturated fats or oils that have gone rancid. When creating a meal plan, it is important for you to be aware of the quality and amount of fats and oils contained in the foods that you will be using. It isn't always easy to identify which foods are high in fat content and which ones aren't. Certain fats are clearly visible. These include margarine, lard, vegetable oil, salad dressing, cream, and butter. Unfortunately, you cannot always tell how much fat a food contains by its appearance. You may be surprised by the large amounts of fat that some foods contain. Some that contain hidden fat include coconuts, avocados, olives, popcorn, nuts, seeds, and various snack foods. Whether you are eating vegetables, fruits, grains, legumes, nuts and seeds, eggs, cheese, or milk, it is a good idea to look for the nutrition information on the package that states the amount of grams of fat per serving.

FAT AND OIL CONTENT OF COMMON FOODS

Like human beings, a seed may have various amounts of fat cells. The percentage of fat or oil in a particular plant will depend on its number of fat cells. Some plants are less than 2 percent fat, while others are as much as 70 percent.

Fruits and Vegetables

Most vegetables—leaves, stems, and roots—have a very low fat content, ranging from a minimum amount of 1 percent fat to a maximum of 8 percent. In the case of dark green leafy vegetables, more than half of their fatty acids are essential in nature and are of very high quality. It is better to eat raw vegetables than cooked ones.

The fat content of fruits is essentially the same as that in vegetables. The only difference is that fruit seeds are high in fat. Fruits contain less linolenic acid than the green parts of plants. People tend to see fruits as more "fattening," since they are higher in sugar than vegetables and will be converted to fat unless you actively burn off these calories.

Grains

Grains are usually made up of 1 to 3 percent fat. About half of the oil in grains contains linoleic acid, so these foods are especially nutritious. When whole grains are used, the oils are stable. However, when a grain is pressed (as in oats), broken (as in steel-cut oats), flaked (as in corn flakes), puffed (as in puffed wheat), popped (as in popcorn), or ground into flour, the oil may spoil rapidly. Boxes of processed grain products that are stored on your cabinet shelf in the summer may go rancid quickly for this reason. When you cook whole grains, the fats remain stable; however, they will begin to deteriorate if the grains are not eaten soon after cooking.

Legumes

Oil content varies more with different legumes than with different grains. As little as 1.1 percent oil comprises lentils and as much as 47.5 percent oil makes up peanuts. Although most people think of peanuts as nuts, they are actually a type of pea. The most desirable of all the legumes are soybeans, both in protein and fat quality, while peanuts are probably the most overrated.

Nuts and Seeds

Nuts and seeds are generally considered to be high in oil, although the range will vary from 1.5 percent for chestnuts to 71.6 percent for macadamia nuts. The oil content in nuts and seeds will vary with the area of growth, the type of fatty acids present, and the yearly climatic changes.

Eggs

For those of you who enjoy eggs for breakfast, you should know that eggs are about 11 percent fat. About 30 percent of the yolk (by weight) consists of fats and oil, while the white of the egg has no fat at all. An egg will contain 250 milligrams of cholesterol! The essential fatty acid content of the yolk will vary depending upon what the chicken has been fed. Free range chickens will produce eggs high in both LA (linoleic acid) and LNA (linolenic acid), while factory farm chickens will contain none.

Cheeses

Although cheeses are good sources of protein, they are generally high in fat and calories as well. Almost without exception, hard cheeses are high in fat. Each gram of fat has nine calories. As in meat, about 50 percent of the fat in cheese is saturated. As much as 33 to 75 percent of the calories in cheese are derived from fat. This high total is clearly undesirable for those who are trying to keep their blood cholesterol levels down.

The rule that hard cheeses are almost always high in fat does have one exception—sapsago, which is generally used for grating. Many dieters will use goat cheese or cheeses that are labeled "part skim" under the mistaken belief that they have a lower fat content than cheeses made from cow's milk. Cheese made from goat's milk has the same fat content as cheese made from cow's milk. Those labeled "part skim" may also have a high fat content if cream has been added.

Milk

Health issues concerning milk involve everything from breastfeeding to cow's milk and goat's milk, and include a variety of nutritional and cultural factors. Approximately 4.4 percent of breast milk is comprised of fat including linoleic acid, gamma linolenic acid (GLA), and small amounts of di-homogamma-linolenic acid (DGLA). Both GLA and DGLA can be converted into arachidonic acid, which is essential for the production of prostaglandins. Neither GLA nor DGLA can be found in most other foods, nor are they present in dairy products. Newborn babies that have been breast-fed will receive prostaglandins that will promote a healthy cardiovascular system. These prostaglandins might be less available for children who haven't been breast-fed. Studies have shown that the fatty acid content of breast milk will vary depending on the diet of the mother. It has been found that the breast milk of mothers who are strict vegetarians is high in linoleic acid yet very low in saturated fatty acids. Interestingly, strict vegetarians have a much lower death rate from cardiovascular disease. Perhaps these statistics are somehow associated with whether they had been breast-fed or whether their mothers were strict vegetarians.

The average fat content of cow's milk is about 3.5 percent, with more than 500 different fatty acids identified in the milk at this time. Many nutritionists do not recommend using cow's milk for a number of reasons. They worry about the harmful effects of formaldehyde, a preservative and carcinogen that is fed to cattle in order to destroy bacteria in the cows' stomachs, which normally would saturate the essential fatty acids that the cows obtain from their food. Many health experts are also concerned about the use of antibiotics and hormones in commercial cattle raising, residues of which may enter the milk.

In various cultures of the world, many different types of milk may be used—milk from camel, sheep, and reindeers, to name a few. In Tibet, yak milk and butter are staples of the diet, and in the United States many people who are allergic to cow's milk or who have a lactose intolerance will use goat's milk instead.

Advances in different cultures have increased the health benefits that can be derived from milk products and have prolonged the time it takes for dairy products to spoil when unrefrigerated. Through bacterial action and the addition of specific bacterial cultures have come products such as yogurt, kefir, buttermilk, and sour cream. This is why sour cream is often labeled "cultured" and yogurt is often described as "containing live cultures." It is recommended that when using cultured milk products, you pick those made from nonfat or part-skim milk.

Fish

The type and quality of fat and fatty acids found in seafood will vary greatly depending on spawning activity, age, season, and variety. While most shellfish are very low in oils, some such as shrimp may be high in cholesterol even when they contain only a moderate fat content. Despite the recent popularity of omega-3 fatty acids, which are found in certain cold-water fish, many nutritionists avoid fish for this reason.

Although much has recently been written about the nutritional benefits of fish, many healers suggest dietary programs that do not include large amounts of fish. Even though fish is low in cholesterol and certainly a superior choice over red meat, present freshwater and salt-water pollution levels and the availability of other sources for all of the essential nutrients at a much lower cost are two reasons that fish is not an essential part of a varied, healthy, and nutritionally balanced program. Since the 1960s there have been warnings about contamination of fish and shellfish by industrial and viral pollutants. Specific warnings have been issued against eating raw freshwater fish or shellfish, and nursing and pregnant women have been advised to avoid freshwater fish.

See Appendix A for a comparison of the fat and cholesterol content of various foods.

READING LABELS FOR FAT CONTENT

Many manufacturers list ingredients and nutritional information on their product labels. Food labels often list calories, protein, carbohydrates, fat, vitamins, and minerals per serving. Manufacturers sometimes list the amount of fiber in products made from grains. Nutritional information can help you choose foods that are high in fiber and vitamins A and C, and also low in fat. Product labels may also list additives and preservatives.

According to the United States Food and Drug Administration, food packages must contain a list of ingredients used in the food product. The ingredients should be listed according to the greatest quantity by weight. With a few exceptions the type of fat contained in a product must be described, so if more than one type of fat is listed and the fat is the first or among the first ingredients listed, you can be sure that the food is high in fat. Even though a food may be low in fat (indicated when fat is one of the last ingredients listed), don't assume that the food will necessarily be beneficial for you, since it is not just the amount of fat that is important to good health, but also the type of fat in the food.

Ingredients on a label are listed in order of prevalence—starting with the ingredient that is used in the greatest amount and ending with the one that is used the least. Whole-wheat bread, for example, might list 100 percent whole-wheat flour as its first ingredient. If a cereal lists sugar first, it means that the cereal contains more sugar than any other ingredient, including grain.

Most processed foods are required to include a panel supplying essential nutritional information about the product. Among the important facts listed on the panel are the number of grams of fat in a specific serving size. The fat content can also be determined by the percentage of calories derived from fats, the grams of saturated and polyunsaturated fats, and the milligrams of cholesterol. When such detailed information is given, the package will probably also state, "Information on fat and cholesterol content is provided for individuals who, on the advice of a physician, are modifying their total dietary intake of fat and/or cholesterol."

A formula has been developed to help you calculate the percentage of calories in a food product that comes from fat. Because there are 9 calories in a gram of fat, the formula is:

$$\frac{? \text{ grams of fat per serving} \times 9 \text{ calories/gram}}{? \text{ total calories per serving}}$$

According to a package label, for example, one serving of peanut butter (the equivalent of 2 tablespoons) contains 16 grams of fat and 200 total calories. Substituting these amounts in our formula, we get:

$$\frac{16 \text{ grams of fat} \times 9 \text{ calories/gram}}{200 \text{ total calories}}$$

To calculate the percentage of fat, multiply 16 grams of fat by 9 calories per gram. Divide the resulting 144 calories by 200 total calories. This equals .72 (or 72 percent). So about 72 percent of the calories in one serving of peanut butter come from fat.

This calculation can be used to identify foods that are higher in fat. To lower your intake of dietary fat, select alternatives containing less fat and either eat smaller amounts of the foods containing more fat or eat them less often. Try to balance your choices of foods that are higher in fat with ones that are lower in fat each day.

CONSUMERS, BEWARE!

Food products are often labeled with appealing descriptive terms such as "lean" or "light" to make them nutritionally appealing. It is hard not to be taken in by them. Commercials are also misleading, and tend to glorify the qualities of a product. The overwhelming number of these food labels and commercials warrants a discussion of them so that you will not misinterpret what the labels actually mean.

Don't Be Fooled by Commercials

A recent letter addressed to the editor of *The New York Times* by a dietician caught my eye, as it questioned the validity of an advertisement. The letter focused on a radio advertisement that issued a true but misleading statement about a line of cold cuts. The advertisement stated that the cold cuts were "99 percent cholesterol free." A dietician pointed out, "That means a serving of three and a half ounces could contain 1,000 milligrams of cholesterol; current recommendations are to eat less than 300 milligrams of cholesterol daily."

Beware of "Lean" and "Lite" Labels

No matter how aware you are of the health risks associated with high-calorie, fatty foods, you may still be fooled by the images that are conjured up by certain food descriptions on labels. Many of these descriptive terms are used by manufacturers to imply that a product is low in fat when they actually mean something else. Among the most misleading and most easily misconstrued terms are "lean," "light," and "extra-light." None of these terms actually means that a product has less calories or fat. Federal law allows these terms to refer to anything from a product's color to its taste and texture. Frozen dinners labeled "lean" will sometimes contain meat and other ingredients that have high levels of fat including palm, palm kernel, and coconut oils. Even though these ingredients are comprised of saturated fats, the law does not require that they be listed specifically on labels.

Don't Be Fooled by Some "Cholesterol-Free" Products

Contrary to the wave of medical claims, many foods that are labeled "cholesterol free" may do more to harden your arteries than the foods they are designed to replace. Unfortunately, the egg substitutes and polyunsaturated margarines that are now heavily marketed are of much lower nutritional value than natural eggs and butter. These substances are composed of artificial colors, flavors, preservatives, and other undesirable ingredients. They also contain trans-fatty acids and other by-products of partial hydrogenation.

MAKING THE RIGHT FOOD CHOICES

As consumers we are constantly bombarded with differing claims about various food products such as butter and margarine, and are presented with many brands of the same food. Are there nutritional differences between butter and margarine, between tub margarines and stick margarines, between gourmet ice creams and ice milk, between different brands of peanut butter, or between air-popped and microwave-popped popcorn? Do some products contain more fat than others? Due to mounting concern about the fat content of foods, the food industry now offers alternatives to many high-fat foods like cheese and ice cream. The problem is finding the ones that are right for you. Read on for some interesting tips on how to make the right food choices.

Cheese

How is cheese manufactured? In cheese production the solids (curds) in milk are coagulated, while the liquids are pressed out. These curds are then solidified by the addition of rennet or some other coagulating agent. Depending on the type of cheese product that is being manufactured, companies will employ different pressing, cooking, and aging techniques. Each pound of cheese may require the use of eight to ten pounds of milk depending on the variety. Most cheeses produced in the United States are made from whole milk, from a combination of whole milk and added cream or skim milk and whole milk, or from a mixture of milk, cream, whey, and skim milk.

Is Pasteurized Process Cheese a Healthy Choice?

Pasteurized process cheese is an interesting invention. In the cheese industry "natural cheese" is a term used to describe pressed curds that have been aged two months or more. (The longer you age the cheese, the sharper it gets.) Pasteurized process cheese is both the best and worst of the processed foods. This product is made from a combination of shredded natural cheeses, mixed with an emulsifier, and then heated to stop the aging process. A positive aspect of this food is that it has less fat than most "natural cheeses," since whey solids, nonfat milk, and water may be added. The higher the amount of these additives, the lower the fat content. Pasteurized process cheese has more additives and less fat than natural cheese. Pasteurized cheese spread has even more additives and less fat than both natural cheese and pasteurized process cheese. Whether these products can really be called cheese at all is questionable; however, if you are concerned about reducing fat, they do have less fat than most cheeses.

The Truth About Ice Cream

In my years as a nutritional consultant, I found that the one food which people were most reluctant to give up was ice cream. Even if their cholesterol levels were sky-high, the thought of going through life without a scoop of double chocolate praline was beyond reason. Is there any hope for the smart consumer who wants to have his ice cream and eat it too? Yes! But you must learn to read labels or it just won't work.

If you were to buy ice cream at a local supermarket back in the 1960s, you could bet that it was filled with artificial flavors and coloring and had about 10 percent fat. (This was the minimum percentage of fat required in a product by the federal government in order for it to be called ice cream.) In recent years new brands of ice cream have come on the market that use higher quality ingredients and have a much richer texture. Unfortunately, these products derive their new texture from an increased fat content. These products, commonly known as "gourmet ice creams," often contain as much as 16 to 20 percent fat by weight. If you are trying to keep your weight down, keep in mind that 50 to 69 percent of the calories in gourmet ice creams are derived from fat. Regular ice creams, various nondairy tofu, and frozen desserts made with vegetable oil are no less fatty. They have simply replaced the butter fat with oil. Despite their levels of saturation, these items still derive from 45 to 55 percent of their calories from fat.

Alternatives to Ice Cream

What are some delicious alternatives to ice cream? There are quite a few! You might enjoy ice milk. Even though it loses some of the creamy texture of high-fat ice cream, ice milk can be a pleasant-tasting replacement. About 25 to 30 percent of its calories come from fat. Or perhaps you might prefer frozen yogurt. This product is often high in sugar, deriving from 8 to 30 percent of its calories from fat. If you are looking for products that do not contain any fat, you might try fruit and juice bars or sorbet. These sweet snacks are generally high in sugar, but have no fat. Many prefer frozen bananas because they have a creamy consistency like ice cream with no fat at all. Simply peel a banana, put it in your freezer, and take it out the next day. You can eat it right out of the freezer, or you can put it through a pulp ejecting juice extracter to create a texture that is closer to that of ice cream.

Food Products Containing Hydrogenated Fats

Research has shown that certain fats containing trans-fatty acids can contribute to an increased rate of cancer. (Refer to Chapter 5 for further information on trans-fatty acids.) These may also be a contributing factor to heart disease and stroke. Trans-fatty acids are a vegetable fat, yet they do not occur naturally in vegetables. How is this possible? The answer is simple—they are manufactured. Many types of snack foods, margarine, salad oils, and mayonnaise contain large amounts of hydrogenated vegetable oil, which has been processed with hydrogen in order to harden the texture and/ or increase the shelf life of the product.

If you are using margarine instead of butter or animal fat to reduce your risk for heart disease, then you may be in for an unpleasant surprise. The total fat content of margarine is high, making it an undesirable choice if you are trying to lower your fat intake.

Margarine: The Good and the Bad

In the 1970s, the number of choices in margarines became overwhelming. It is not surprising that consumers are often confused about both the benefits of margarine over butter and the differences from brand to brand. Among the types of margarine products available are hard margarine in stick form, liquid margarine in bottles, soft margarine in tubs, and margarine made from different oils (primarily cottonseed, sunflower, corn, and soybean).

Margarine is popular for a number of reasons. Many use margarine because its health benefits are considered greater than those derived from butter, and it is generally less costly. In addition, margarine contains more of the polyunsaturated oils that are known to lower blood cholesterol levels than butter. A big plus is that margarine doesn't have any cholesterol.

Comparing Margarine Products

When buying margarine, it is important to make comparisons based on the ratio of polyunsaturated to saturated fat, the aroma, the type of oil used, the caloric and sodium content, as well as the price and taste. In order to make a wise choice, however, you *must* consider the amount of polyunsaturated fat that the margarine contains. The softer the margarine is, the more desirable it will be, since it will cover a slice of bread more easily and thus enable you to cut down on your caloric consumption. Many avoid using butter or margarine in stick form on breads because it is harder to spread and tends to tear bread. Although some tub margarines are softer than others, this difference disappears once they have been out of the refrigerator for thirty minutes or more. For individuals with hypertension, it is important to use salt-free margarines.

For Cooking

Whether you are using regular, stick, or tub margarines or a margarine/butter blend, you can fry or bake with them the same as you can with butter. The margarines that contain milk products, however, will burn more quickly than the margarines made solely from oil. Reduced-calorie margarines cannot be substituted for regular margarine or butter in baking since they are much lower in fat (due to their high water content), and would produce baked goods that are too hard. These margarines are also more difficult to use in frying, though few product labels will tell you so. Many margarine products will display the words "no cholesterol" on the front of the package. This is about as useful as putting a no cholesterol label on frozen spinach, since neither frozen spinach nor margarine would contain cholesterol anyway.

Some people on weight-reduction programs use margarines under the mistaken belief that they have less calories
than butter. This is not true. There is no direct connection
between the amount of calories in margarine and the level of
saturated fat. In fact, margarines having less calories may
sometimes be higher in saturated fat. It is especially important to keep this in mind when purchasing butter/margarine
blends.

For Fat Content

It is important for you to evaluate the ratio of polyunsaturated fats to saturated fats when deciding which margarines
will promote good nutrition. For example, if a margarine
contains twice as much polyunsaturated fat as saturated fat,
it is desirable, since it takes twice as much polyunsaturated
fat to effect a cholesterol reduction in your blood. The majority of margarines will list this ratio on the label. In fact, they
will often use larger numbers than necessary when listing
this ratio (4 to 2 instead of 2 to 1) in an attempt to make their
product seem more desirable. Of all the available margarines, the tub margarines seem to have the best ratio—as
much as 2.5 to 1 of polyunsaturated to saturated fat. The
reason for this difference is a simple one. Tub margarines
contain less hydrogenated oil than stick margarines. In fact,
it is the hydrogenation process—the means by which the oil
is hardened—that converts unsaturated fat into saturated
fat. For this reason, it is always better to avoid the stick
margarines.

If you are not particularly adept at label reading, especially concerning the ratios described above, you may be
able to obtain all you need to know simply by looking at the
list of ingredients. Those margarines with a higher level of
unsaturated fat will generally have liquid oil as their first ingredient. Food and Drug Administration standards for the
fat content of margarine are about the same as those for butter. They require that margarine contain 80 percent fat.
Thus, *both* regular margarine and butter will contain at least

100 calories per tablespoon. While butter may contain a higher level of fat that is ingested than margarine, switching to margarine will neither help you to lose weight nor to lower overall fat consumption. Many nutritionists and physicians feel that it is more important to lower overall fat consumption than to focus on increasing unsaturated fats and reducing saturated fats. Products known as "spreads" and "imitation" margarines will contain from 50 to 90 calories per tablespoon.

Although all margarines consist primarily of oil, other ingredients include nonfat milk solids, water, or whey. Other ingredients such as lecithin and mono- and diglycerides will be added to keep the water and oil from separating. The lecithin is also valuable in keeping the margarine from splattering during frying. Other chemicals such as potassium sorbate, citric acid, sodium benzoate, and calcium disodium EDTA may be used as preservatives in margarine. Most natural foods enthusiasts and nutritionists will avoid margarine products that contain these chemicals, especially since there are margarines available in health food stores that use naturally derived preservatives as antioxidants.

Most commercial brands of margarine also add artificial color and flavor to make the products appear more like butter. (These chemicals may also be added to butter during the winter months.) All margarines must be fortified with vitamin D as a result of federal law.

Natural Peanut Butter Versus Peanut Butter With Hydrogenated Oil

Although peanut butter has tradionally been viewed as a favorite food among children, a "recent industry survey shows that adults make up almost 50% of the peanut butter-eating public." Much of this adult consumption includes the gourmet varieties that contain bananas, chocolate, and marshmallows.

The fat content of different peanut butters does not change even when they contain sugar and other additives.

Peanut butter, like all other bean products (that's right, a peanut is a bean—not a nut), does not contain cholesterol. It contains approximately eight grams of fat per tablespoon. Each tablespoon may contain as much as eighty calories, 70 percent of which come from fat. Most commercial peanut butter products may contain up to 10 percent hydrogenated vegetable oil (usually added as an emulsifier to keep the peanut oil from separating), salt, and sweeteners including molasses, dextrose, sugar, and corn syrup. Artificial flavorings, artificial sweeteners, chemical preservatives, vitamins, and colorings are never added to peanut butter because it is prohibited by law.

Most of the fat in peanut butter is monounsaturated and polyunsaturated. The hydrogenated oil that is often added does not greatly increase the very small amount of saturated fat that occurs. In its natural state (without additives), peanut butter is a nutritionally sound food, containing such minerals as calcium, iron, phosphorus, potassium, and zinc, as well as B vitamins. Freshly ground peanut butter can be purchased in most health food stores. It contains nothing but fresh roasted peanuts and salt. Because no hydrogenated fats have been added to this product, you can reduce the fat content by removing the oil when it separates. When its oil has been removed, however, the peanut butter may lose some of its taste since it gets much of its flavor from the oil.

In recent years it has been discovered that certain toxic molds, called aflatoxins, can form on peanuts under certain conditions. As long as peanut growers are conscientious and monitor their crops, this does not seem to pose a problem.

If you are a peanut butter lover, you may be interested in the following bits of information:

- There is no nutritional difference between chunky and smooth varieties.

- Women prefer chunky while men are evenly divided between chunky and smooth (according to the Peanut Advisory Board).

- Most natural brands contain about 5 to 9 percent natural sugar, while commercial brands with added sugar may contain as much as 14 percent of the sweetener.

- Each tablespoon of peanut butter contains approximately 100 calories.

Other Ground Nut and Seed Butters as Alternatives

With the popularity of peanut butter growing daily, many people have developed an interest in other nut and seed butters such as almond, sunflower, and sesame butter. Sesame tahini, a very popular food in the Middle East, is a rich paste made from ground sesame seeds and is generally found in Greek, Armenian, and health food stores.

Popcorn

Popcorn prepared in a hot-air popping machine can be a nutritious, high-fiber snack food that is low in both salt and fat. Unpopped corn is now available for microwave popping; this innovation can be a saturated fat nightmare. Popping with oil (usually soybean, cottonseed, palm, or palm kernel) can increase the fat content of the popcorn to 1.4 grams and bring its calorie count to more than 100 calories per serving. Read your labels.

Fruit Juices and Drinks

Oils that have been treated with bromine are often added to processed juice drinks to keep them from becoming cloudy and to prevent juice rings from forming in the bottle necks. They are added solely for cosmetic effect. Unfortunately, brominated oils, which are generally made from cottonseed, soybeans, corn, sesame, and olives, can cause changes in essential organs and tissues including the thyroid gland, kidney, liver, and heart. Brominated oils have also been shown to cause a withering of the testicles. The danger of brominated oils has been so clearly demonstrated that they have been banned from fruit juices and drinks in Germany and Holland.

THE HEALTHY HEART SEAL OF APPROVAL

In June 1988 the American Heart Association (AHA) announced its intentions to identify and endorse processed foods that meet its dietary guidelines. In particular these guidelines will assess the cholesterol, fat, and salt content of foods. AHA has indicated that an independent testing group will evaluate margarines, cooking oils, and salad dressings first for possible approval. This seal of approval will be given primarily to processed foods. This is a good step forward, however, it does not seem as if the AHA will take into account the role of artificial ingredients, flavorings, chemicals, and other factors in heart disease.

GOVERNMENT GRADING OF BEEF: MAKING SENSE OF IT ALL

Every few years we are presented with a new system for grading beef. These changes are primarily the result of various lobbying efforts. When the cattle farmers are particularly effective, higher fat content is touted for its marbling and for its fuller flavor. When the consumer lobby is stronger, you will hear of the benefits of lean beef. Essentially you can have a well-balanced diet that does not include beef. If, however, you intend to use beef in your diet, you may be interested in its history and the new USDA labels.

It would be helpful for you to know the qualifications a cut of meat would have to meet in order to be given a certain label. For example, a meat identified as "extra lean" means that it is no more than 5 percent fat. Those cuts that are labeled by the USDA as "lean" (also called low fat) can be comprised of no more than 10 percent fat. Foods identified as "light" (also called "lite," "leaner," and "low fat") earn their labels by containing 25 percent less fat than the majority of such products on the market.

You should also be aware of changes in the way meats are graded. Slightly marbled beef, previously graded as "USDA Good," is now being graded as "USDA select," while the leanest type of beef that was previously graded "good" has now been upgraded to the more appealing "select." Beef purchased from your local supermarket is graded by the USDA from most to least marbled; it is labeled either as prime, choice, or select.

If all of these identifications are confusing, then let's add more fat to the fire (so to speak). Unlike "lean beef," "lean" ground beef is allowed to contain as much as 22.5 percent fat. This amount is more than double the 10 percent fat allowed for a cut of "lean beef."

FOOD ADDITIVES

When a chemical agent or a mixture of substances (natural or synthetic) is added to a food during any phase of manufacturing, storage, or packaging, it is generally called an "additive." Some additives come from natural sources, but a great number of additives are synthesized from petroleum or coal-tar derivatives. These additives are generally cheap replacements for ingredients that would otherwise enhance flavor and texture, add stability, improve nutritional value, prevent separation (fats and water do not mix), and retard spoilage.

Some additives are used in food to reduce the effects of oxidation. Certain foods will spoil when exposed to air. Signs of spoilage include discoloration or flavor change. When you cut certain foods such as apples and peaches, you will notice that the exposed surface turns brown. These changes occur when these foods are exposed to oxygen. By adding various antioxidants to food products, color changes due to oxidation are minimized. Among the most commonly used antioxidants in process foods are butylated hydroxyanisole (BHA), butylated hydroxytoluene (BHT), and propyl gallate.

Certain liquids just will not mix. You know about oil and water. You can shake them, blend them, and mix them, but if you wait a few minutes, the oil will rise to the top. This can be a problem if you're trying to bake cake or bread. There are certain agents that can be added to liquids that ordinarily would not mix, which would cause them to blend and remain stable or "emulsify." Eggs were probably one of the first "emulsifying agents." In fact, the use of eggs in cooking has enabled people to mix fats, watery liquids, and air to add a lighter texture to baked goods. Emulsification has been found especially useful in keeping the oil blended in foods such as frozen desserts, pourable salad dressings, ice cream, and chocolate. Ice cream would not have its uniform, smooth texture if it weren't for the emulsifiers that permit the complete blending of ingredients. Among the most commonly used emulsifiers in processed foods are lecithin (a soybean derivative) and mono- and diglycerides.

Eating can be enjoyable and nutritious if you choose the right foods in the right amounts. Fats and oils are necessary for good health; however, you have seen how you must beware of misleading advertising and labels and limit your use of products that contain too much fat. If you use this book as a reference text on a regular basis and follow its recommendations, you will have the tools for reducing your risk of cancer, cardiovascular disease, stroke, heart attack, and many other diseases. Fats and oils are essential to life, and if used properly and effectively, they can help you heal and build and maintain a healthy lifestyle.

Afterword

In February of 1990, investigators from the National Cholesterol Education Program, a blue-ribbon federal health panel, released an important report on the pressing need to reduce our daily intake of fat. This panel, which was made up of thirty-eight public and private health organizations ranging from the American Heart Association to the American Medical Association, strongly recommended that all Americans limit the number of calories derived from fat to no more than 30 percent of their daily diet. At almost the same time, the Food and Drug Administration approved the first substitute fat for United States consumption. The product, Simplesse, is manufactured by the NutraSweet Company, a subsidiary of the giant St. Louis-based chemical firm Monsanto Company. Simplesse is made by cooking the proteins found in egg whites and milk, and then blending them into a fluid that has the texture and taste of fat, but fewer calories and no cholesterol. It replaces fat, at nine calories per gram, with protein, at four calories per gram. Because Simplesse cannot be baked or fried without losing its creamy texture, it has been approved for use only in frozen desserts at this time.

Waiting in the wings for future FDA approval are a host of other less-than-natural fake fats, such as Olestra, a product developed by Procter & Gamble. While Olestra exhibits almost all of the characteristics of real fat, it cannot be digested or absorbed by our bodies. Kraft is testing a product that is similar to Simplesse, but which the company hopes will be a substitute cooking fat with absolutely no calories or cholesterol.

It would seem that the development and release of these fake fats could not come at a more opportune time for immediate public acceptance. Once a number of these substitute fat products gain FDA approval, their proliferated use in commercially prepared foods will be nothing more than astounding. While these seemingly fantastic breakthroughs will be heralded by the media, the more unsettling question to be asked is, at what price?

There are three major points to consider regarding the use of fake fats. First, will these products serve a useful purpose? For people who absolutely don't care about what they eat, but don't want to be overweight, fake fats will be a miracle product. It will enable them to continue eating a new variety of the "Great American Diet" made up of substantially less fat-derived calories. It also will most likely be recommended to patients suffering from high blood pressure, heart diseases, and excess weight problems by mainstream physicians and nutritionists. The use of fake fat is likely to result in weight loss and better weight maintenance.

Second, will there be any harmful effects directly linked to the eating of these fat substitutes? Currently, there is no hard evidence to suggest that ingesting these products will cause any terrible allergic reactions or diseases for the vast majority of consumers. However, while I am not trying to be an alarmist, recent history tells us that the more a "food" is refined or created out of nonfood-generated chemicals, and the greater quantities we eat of these products, the less likely it is that the "food" will add to our general well-being. The sad fact is that these products' negative side effects may take years to be uncovered.

Third, will there be any indirect harmful effects caused by fat substitutes? The answer is a resounding yes. In the long run, the growing use of fake fats will have a devastating effect on our health. Over the last twenty years, the wholistic movement in our country has strived to point out how nutritionally poor our "modern diet" of fast foods and convenience foods is. The links between the foods we eat and this nation's two top killer diseases, heart disease and cancer, have now been firmly established. However, with the future availability of "fat-less" foods, the vast majority of people will continue to eat an imbalanced, nutritionally poor diet.

Instead of replacing hamburgers with fish, fried potatoes with fresh vegetables, or ice cream with fruit, we will now be tempted to consume the "fat-less" burgers, fries, and ice cream that contain less fat-derived calories. Why eat highly nutritious, high-fiber, fresh whole foods when we can still have our standard over-salted, over-sugared, over-refined favorites? The fact is that these new products will allow us to keep our heads in the sand just a bit longer—until we discover that we have lost our health, and that we had better take a closer look at what proper nutrition means.

The point is simple. The ultimate responsibility of what we eat is ours. If we wish to be influenced by high-impact commercials, pretty packaging, or financially motivated fads, that is our right. If we wish to add a little more reason to our diet, that too is our right. We should, however, always consider the consequences of the choices we make on ourselves and our families.

The purpose of this book is to give you a better idea of how important real fats and oils are in your life, and what you can do to make the best of what is available to you. The fact that you have read this book indicates that you are on your way to making the right decisions.

Appendices

Appendix A
Fat and Cholesterol Content of Foods

The following tables list the fat and cholesterol content of different foods. Food groups included are dairy products; nuts and seeds; breads, cereals, pasta, rice, and dried peas and beans; meats; poultry; fish; sweets and snacks; and other miscellaneous foods. When planning your meals, try to choose items listed at the beginning of each group to lower your fat and cholesterol levels. Note that the fat and cholesterol content of the product listed will vary slightly from sample to sample. The fat and cholesterol content of the food product tested will vary according to individual differences between animals (based upon their diets and exercise), the part of the animal being tested, and/or the way in which the food product was manufactured or processed.

The nutritional information for the foods listed in this appendix is based on publications of the United States Department of Agriculture.

Fat and Cholesterol Content of Dairy Products

Product	Saturated Fat (Grams)	Cholesterol (Milligrams)	Total Fat[1] (Grams)	Calories from Fat[2](%)	Total Calories
Milk (8 ounces)					
Skim milk	0.3	4	0.4	5	86
Buttermilk	1.3	9	2.2	20	99
Low-fat milk, 1% fat	1.6	10	2.6	23	102
Low-fat milk, 2% fat	2.9	18	4.7	35	121
Whole milk, 3.3% fat	5.1	33	8.2	49	150
Yogurt (4 ounces)					
Plain yogurt, low fat	0.1	2	0.2	3	63
Plain yogurt	2.4	14	3.7	47	70
Cheese					
Cottage cheese, low-fat, 1% fat, 4 oz.	0.7	5	1.2	13	82
Mozzarella, part-skim, 1 oz.	2.9	16	4.5	56	72
Cottage cheese, creamed, 4 oz.	3.2	17	5.1	39	117
Mozzarella, 1 oz.	3.7	22	6.1	69	80
Sour cream, 1 oz.	3.7	12	5.9	87	61
American processed cheese spread, pasteurized, 1 oz.	3.8	16	6.0	66	82
Feta, 1 oz.	4.2	25	6.0	72	75
Neufchâtel, 1 oz.	4.2	22	6.6	81	74
Camembert, 1 oz.	4.3	20	6.9	73	85
American processed cheese food, pasteurized, 1 oz.	4.4	18	7.0	68	93
Provolone, 1 oz.	4.8	20	7.6	68	100
Limburger, 1 oz.	4.8	26	7.7	75	93
Brie, 1 oz.	4.9	28	7.9	74	95

Fat and Cholesterol Content of Dairy Products—*Continued*

Product	Saturated Fat (Grams)	Cholesterol (Milligrams)	Total Fat[1] (Grams)	Calories from Fat[2](%)	Total Calories
Romano, 1 oz.	4.9	29	7.6	63	110
Gouda, 1 oz.	5.0	32	7.8	69	101
Swiss, 1 oz.	5.0	26	7.8	65	107
Edam, 1 oz.	5.0	25	7.9	70	101
Brick, 1 oz.	5.3	27	8.4	72	105
Blue, 1 oz.	5.3	21	8.2	73	100
Gruyère, 1 oz.	5.4	31	9.2	71	117
Muenster, 1 oz.	5.4	27	8.5	74	104
Parmesan, 1 oz.	5.4	22	8.5	59	129
Monterey Jack, 1 oz.	5.5	25	8.6	73	106
Roquefort, 1 oz.	5.5	26	8.7	75	105
Ricotta, part-skim, 4 oz.	5.6	25	9.0	52	156
American processed cheese, pasteurized, 1 oz.	5.6	27	8.9	75	106
Colby, 1 oz.	5.7	27	9.1	73	112
Cheddar, 1 oz.	6.0	30	9.4	74	114
Cream cheese, 1 oz.	6.2	31	9.9	90	99
Ricotta, whole milk, 4 oz.	9.4	58	14.7	67	197
Eggs					
Egg, chicken, white	0	0	tr.	0	16
Egg, chicken, whole	1.7	274	5.6	64	79
Egg, chicken, yolk	1.7	272	5.6	80	63

[1]Total fat = saturated fatty acids plus monounsaturated fatty acids plus polyunsaturated fatty acids.

[2]Percent calories from fat = (total fat calories divided by total calories) multiplied by 100; total fat calories = total fat (grams) multiplied by 9.

oz. = ounce
tr. = trace

Source: *Composition of Foods: Dairy and Egg Products—Raw * Processed * Prepared, Agriculture Handbook 8-1*. United States Department of Agriculture, Agricultural Research Service (November 1976).

Fat and Cholesterol Content of Nuts and Seeds

Product (1 Ounce	Saturated Fatty Acids (Grams)	Cholesterol (Milligrams)	Total Fat[1] (Grams)	Calories from Fat[2](%)	Total Calories
European chestnuts	0.2	0	1.1	9	105
Filberts or hazelnuts	1.3	0	17.8	89	179
Almonds	1.4	0	15.0	80	167
Pecans	1.5	0	18.4	89	187
Sunflower seed kernels, roasted	1.5	0	1.4	77	165
English walnuts	1.6	0	17.6	87	182
Pistachio nuts	1.7	0	13.7	75	164
Peanuts	1.9	0	14.0	76	164
Hickory nuts	2.0	0	18.3	88	187
Pine nuts, pignolia	2.2	0	14.4	89	146
Pumpkin and squash seed kernels	2.3	0	12.0	73	148
Cashew nuts	2.6	0	13.2	73	163
Macadamia nuts	3.1	0	20.9	95	199
Brazil nuts	4.6	0	18.8	91	186
Coconut meat, unsweetened	16.3	0	18.3	88	187

[1]Total fat = saturated fatty acids plus monounsaturated fatty acids plus polyunsaturated fatty acids.

[2]Percent calories from fat = (total fat calories divided by total calories) multiplied by 100; total fat calories = total fat (grams) multiplied by 9.

Sources: *Composition of Foods: Legumes and Legume Products—Raw * Processed * Prepared, Agriculture Handbook 8-16.* United States Department of Agriculture, Human Nutrition Information Service (December 1986).

*Composition of Foods: Nut and Seed Products—Raw * Processed * Prepared, Agriculture Handbook 8-12.* United States Department of Agriculture, Human Nutrition Information Service (September 1984).

Fat and Cholesterol Content of Breads, Cereals, Pasta, Rice, and Dried Peas and Beans

Product	Saturated Fatty Acids (Grams)	Cholesterol (Milligrams)	Total Fat[1] (Grams)	Calories from Fat[2] (%)	Total Calories
Breads					
Melba toast, 1 plain	0.1	0	tr.	0	20
Pita, ½ large shell	0.1	0	1.0	5	165
Corn tortilla	0.1	0	1.0	14	65
Rye bread, 1 slice	0.2	0	1.0	14	65
English muffin	0.3	0	1.0	6	140
Bagel, 1, 3½" diameter	0.3	0	2.0	9	200
Rye krisp, 2 triple crackers	0.3	0	1.0	16	56
Whole wheat bread, 1 slice	0.4	0	1.0	13	70
Saltines, 4	0.5	4	1.0	18	50
Hamburger bun	0.5	tr.	2.0	16	115
Hot dog bun	0.5	tr.	2.0	16	115
Pancake, 1, 4" diameter	0.5	16	2.0	30	60
Bran muffin, 1, 2½" diameter	1.4	24	6.0	43	125
Corn muffin, 1, 2½" diameter	1.5	23	5.0	31	145
Plain doughnut, 1, 3¼" diameter	2.8	20	12.0	51	210
Croissant, 1, 4½" by 4"	3.5	13	12.0	46	235
Waffle, 1, 7" diameter	4.0	102	13.0	48	245
Cereals (1 cup)					
Corn flakes	tr.	—	0.1	0	98
Cream of wheat, cooked	tr.	—	0.5	3	134
Corn grits, cooked	tr.	—	0.5	3	146
Oatmeal, cooked	0.4	—	2.4	15	145
Granola	5.8	—	33.1	50	595
100% Natural Cereal with raisins and dates	13.7	—	20.3	37	496

Fat and Cholesterol Content of Breads, Cereals, Pasta, Rice, and Dried Peas and Beans—*Continued*

Product	Saturated Fatty Acids (Grams)	Cholesterol (Milligrams)	Total Fat[1] (Grams)	Calories from Fat[2](%)	Total Calories
Pasta (1 cup)					
Spaghetti, cooked	0.1	0	1.0	6	155
Elbow macaroni, cooked	0.1	0	1.0	6	155
Egg noodles, cooked	0.5	50	2.0	11	160
Chow mein noodles, canned	2.1	5	11.0	45	220
Rice (1 cup cooked)					
Rice, white	0.1	0	0.5	2	225
Rice, brown	0.3	0	1.0	4	230
Dried Peas and Beans (1 cup cooked)					
Split peas	0.1	0	0.8	3	231
Kidney beans	0.1	0	1.0	4	225
Lima beans	0.2	0	0.7	3	217
Black eyed peas	0.3	0	1.2	5	200
Garbanzo beans	0.4	0	4.3	14	269

[1]Total fat = saturated fatty acids plus monounsaturated fatty acids plus polyunsaturated fatty acids.

[2]Percent calories from fat = (total fat calories divided by total calories) multiplied by 100; total fat calories = total fat (grams) multiplied by 9.

— = information not available in sources used.

oz. = ounce

tr. = trace

Sources: *Composition of Foods: Breakfast Cereals—Raw * Processed * Prepared, Agriculture Handbook 8-8.* United States Department of Agriculture, Human Nutrition Information Service (July 1982).

Composition of Foods: Legume and Legume Products, Agriculture Handbook 8-16. United States Department of Agriculture, Nutrition Monitoring Division (December 1986).

Home and Garden Bulletin. Nutritive Value of Foods. No. 72. United States Department of Agriculture. Human Nutrition Information Service (1986).

Fat and Cholesterol Content of Meats

Product (3½ Ounces, Cooked)*	Saturated Fatty Acids (Grams)	Cholesterol (Milligrams)	Total Fat[1] (Grams)	Calories from Fat[2](%)	Total Calories
Beef					
Kidneys, simmered[3]	1.1	387	3.4	21	144
Liver, braised[3]	1.9	389	4.9	27	161
Round, top round, lean only, broiled	2.2	84	6.2	29	191
Round, eye of round, lean only, roasted	2.5	69	6.5	32	183
Round, tip round, lean only, roasted	2.8	81	7.5	36	190
Round, full cut, lean only, choice, broiled	2.9	82	8.0	37	194
Round, bottom round, lean only, braised	3.4	96	9.7	39	222
Short loin, top loin, lean only, broiled	3.6	76	8.9	40	203
Wedge-bone sirloin, lean only, broiled	3.6	89	8.7	38	208
Short loin, tenderloin, lean only, broiled	3.6	84	9.3	41	204
Chuck, arm pot roast, lean only, braised	3.8	101	10.0	39	231
Short loin, T-bone steak, lean only, choice, broiled	4.2	80	10.4	44	214

Fat and Cholesterol Content of Meats—*Continued*

Product (3½ Ounces, Cooked)*	Saturated Fatty Acids (Grams)	Cholesterol (Milligrams)	Total Fat[1] (Grams)	Calories from Fat[2](%)	Total Calories
Short loin, porterhouse steak, lean only, choice, broiled	4.3	80	10.8	45	218
Brisket, whole, lean only, braised	4.6	93	12.8	48	241
Rib eye, small (ribs 10-12), lean only, choice, broiled	4.9	80	11.6	47	225
Rib, whole (ribs 6-12), lean only, roasted	5.8	81	13.8	52	240
Flank, lean only, choice, braised	5.9	71	13.8	51	244
Rib, large end (ribs 6-9), lean only, broiled	6.1	82	14.2	55	233
Chuck, blade roast, lean only, braised	6.2	106	15.3	51	270
Corned beef, cured, brisket, cooked	6.3	98	19.0	68	251
Flank, lean and fat, choice, braised	6.6	72	15.5	54	257
Ground, lean, broiled medium	7.2	87	18.5	61	272
Round, full cut, lean and fat, choice, braised	7.3	84	18.2	60	274
Rib, short ribs, lean only, choice, braised	7.7	93	18.1	55	295

Product (3½ Ounces, Cooked)*	Saturated Fatty Acids (Grams)	Cholesterol (Milligrams)	Total Fat[1] (Grams)	Calories from Fat[2](%)	Total Calories
Salami, cured, cooked, smoked, 3-4 slices	9.0	65	20.7	71	262
Short loin, T-bone steak, lean and fat, choice, broiled	10.2	84	24.6	68	324
Chuck, arm pot roast, lean and fat, braised	10.7	99	26.0	67	350
Sausage, cured, cooked, smoked, about 2	11.4	67	26.9	78	312
Bologna, cured, 3-4 slices	12.1	58	28.5	82	312
Frankfurter, cured, about 2	12.0	61	28.5	82	315
Lamb					
Leg, lean only, roast, lean and fat, braised	3.0	89	8.2	39	191
Loin chop, lean only, broiled	4.1	94	9.4	39	215
Rib, lean only, roasted	5.7	88	12.3	48	232
Arm chop, lean only, braised	6.0	122	14.6	47	279
Rib, lean and fat, roasted	14.2	90	30.6	75	368
Pork					
Cured, ham steak, boneless, extra lean, unheated	1.4	45	4.2	31	122
Liver, braised[3]	1.4	355	4.4	24	165
Kidneys, braised[3]	1.5	480	4.7	28	151

Fat and Cholesterol Content of Meats—*Continued*

Product (3½ Ounces, Cooked)*	Saturated Fatty Acids (Grams)	Cholesterol (Milligrams)	Total Fat[1] (Grams)	Calories from Fat[2](%)	Total Calories
Fresh, loin, tenderloin, lean only, roasted	1.7	93	4.8	26	166
Cured, shoulder, arm picnic, lean only, roasted	2.4	48	7.0	37	170
Cured, ham, boneless, regular, roasted	3.1	59	9.0	46	178
Fresh, leg (ham), shank half, lean only, roasted	3.6	92	10.5	44	215
Fresh, leg (ham), rump half, lean only, roasted	3.7	96	10.7	43	221
Fresh, loin, center loin, sirloin, lean only, roasted	4.5	91	13.1	49	240
Fresh, loin, sirloin, lean only, roasted	4.5	90	13.2	50	236
Fresh, loin, center rib, lean only, roasted	4.8	79	13.8	51	245
Fresh, loin, top loin, lean only, roasted	4.8	79	13.8	51	245
Fresh, shoulder, blade, Boston, lean only, roasted	5.8	98	16.8	59	256
Fresh, loin, blade, lean only, roasted	6.6	89	19.3	62	279

Product (3½ Ounces, Cooked)*	Saturated Fatty Acids (Grams)	Cholesterol (Milligrams)	Total Fat[1] (Grams)	Calories from Fat[2](%)	Total Calories
Fresh, loin, sirloin, lean and fat, roasted	7.4	91	20.4	63	291
Cured, shoulder, arm picnic, lean and fat, roasted	7.7	58	21.4	69	280
Fresh, loin, center loin, lean and fat, roasted	7.9	91	21.8	64	305
Cured, shoulder, blade roll, lean and fat, roasted	8.4	67	23.5	74	287
Fresh, Italian sausage, cooked	9.0	78	25.7	72	323
Fresh, bratwurst, cooked	9.3	60	25.9	77	301
Fresh, chitterlings, cooked	10.1	143	28.8	86	303
Cured, liver sausage, liverwurst	10.6	158	28.5	79	326
Cured, smoked link sausage, grilled	11.3	68	31.8	74	389
Fresh, spareribs, lean and fat, braised	11.8	121	30.3	69	397
Cured, salami, dry or hard	11.9	—	33.7	75	407
Bacon, fried	17.4	85	49.2	78	576
Veal					
Rump, lean only, roasted	—	128	2.2	13	156
Sirloin, lean only, roasted	—	128	3.2	19	153

Fat and Cholesterol Content of Meats—*Continued*

Product (3½ Ounces, Cooked)*	Saturated Fatty Acids (Grams)	Cholesterol (Milligrams)	Total Fat[1] (Grams)	Calories from Fat[2](%)	Total Calories
Arm steak, lean only, cooked	—	90	5.3	24	200
Loin chop, lean only, cooked	—	90	6.7	29	207
Blade, lean only, cooked	—	90	7.8	33	211
Cutlet, medium fat, braised or broiled	4.8	128	11.0	37	271
Foreshank, medium fat, stewed	—	90	10.4	43	216
Plate, medium fat, stewed	—	90	21.2	63	303
Rib, medium fat, roasted	7.1	128	16.9	70	218
Flank, medium fat, stewed	—	90	32.3	75	390

*3½ ozs = 100 grams (approximately).

[1]Total fat = saturated fatty acids plus monounsaturated fatty acids plus polyunsaturated fatty acids.

[2]Percent calories from fat = (total fat calories divided by total calories) multiplied by 100; total fat calories = total fat (grams) multiplied by 9.

[3]Liver and most organ meats are low in fat, but high in cholesterol. If you are eating to lower your blood cholesterol, you should consider your total cholesterol intake before selecting an organ meat.

— = information not available in sources used.

Sources: *Composition of Foods: Beef Products—Raw * Processed * Prepared, Agriculture Handbook 8-13*. United States Department of Agriculture, Human Nutrition Information Service (August 1986).

*Composition of Foods: Pork Products—Raw * Processed * Prepared, Agriculture Handbook 8-10*. United States Department of Agriculture, Human Nutrition Information Service (August 1983).

Home and Garden Bulletin. Nutritive Value of Foods. No. 72. United States Department of Agriculture. Human Nutrition Information Service (1986).

Fat and Cholesterol Content of Poultry

Product (3½ Ounces, Cooked)*	Saturated Fatty Acids (Grams)	Cholesterol (Milligrams)	Total Fat[1] (Grams)	Calories from Fat[2](%)	Total Calories
Turkey, fryer-roasters, light meat without skin, roasted	0.4	86	1.9	8	140
Chicken, roasters, light meat without skin, roasted	1.1	75	4.1	24	153
Turkey, fryer-roasters, light meat with skin, roasted	1.3	95	4.6	25	164
Chicken, broilers or fryers, light meat without skin, roasted	1.3	85	4.5	24	173
Turkey, fryer-roasters, dark meat without skin, roasted	1.4	112	4.3	24	162
Chicken, stewing, light meat without skin, stewed	2.0	70	8.0	34	213
Turkey roll, light and dark	2.0	55	7.0	42	149
Turkey, fryer-roasters, dark meat with skin, roasted	2.1	117	7.1	35	182
Chicken, roasters, dark meat without skin, roasted	2.4	75	8.8	44	178
Chicken, broilers or fryers, dark meat without skin, roasted	2.7	93	9.7	43	205
Chicken, broilers or fryers, light meat with skin, roasted	3.0	85	10.9	44	222

Fat and Cholesterol Content of Poultry—*Continued*

Product (3½ Ounces, Cooked)*	Saturated Fatty Acids (Grams)	Cholesterol (Milligrams)	Total Fat[1] (Grams)	Calories from Fat[2](%)	Total Calories
Chicken, stewing, dark meat without skin, stewed	4.1	95	15.3	53	258
Duck, domesticated, flesh only, roasted	4.2	89	11.2	50	201
Chicken, broilers or fryers, dark meat with skin, roasted	4.4	91	15.8	56	253
Goose, domesticated, flesh only, roasted	4.6	96	12.7	48	238
Turkey bologna, about 3½ slices	5.1	99	15.2	69	199
Chicken frank-furter, about 2	5.5	101	19.5	68	257
Turkey frank-furter, about 2	5.9	107	17.7	70	226

*3½ ozs = 100 grams (approximately).

[1]Total fat = saturated fatty acids plus monounsaturated fatty acids plus polyunsaturated fatty acids.

[2]Percent calories from fat = (total fat calories divided by total calories) multiplied by 100; total fat calories = total fat (grams) multiplied by 9.

Source: *Composition of Foods: Poultry Products—Raw * Processed * Prepared, Agriculture Handbook 8-5*. United States Department of Agriculture, Science and Education Administration (August 1979).

Fat and Cholesterol Content of Fish

Product (3½ Ounces, Cooked)*	Saturated Fatty Acids (Grams)	Cholesterol (Milligrams)	Omega-3 Fatty Acids (Grams)	Total Fat[1] (Grams)	Calories from Fat[2](%)	Total Calories
Finfish						
Haddock, dry heat	0.2	74	0.2	0.9	7	112
Cod, Atlantic, dry heat	0.2	55	0.2	0.9	7	105
Pollock, walleye, dry heat	0.2	96	1.5	1.1	9	113
Perch, mixed species, dry heat	0.2	42	0.3	1.2	9	117
Grouper, mixed species, dry heat	0.3	47	—	1.3	10	118
Whiting, mixed species, dry heat	0.3	84	0.9	1.7	13	115
Snapper, mixed species, dry heat	0.4	47	—	1.7	12	128
Halibut, Atlantic and Pacific, dry heat	0.4	41	0.6	2.9	19	140
Rockfish, Pacific, dry heat	0.5	44	0.5	2.0	15	121
Sea bass, mixed species, dry heat	0.7	53	—	2.5	19	124
Trout, rainbow, dry heat	0.8	73	0.9	4.3	26	151
Swordfish, dry heat	1.4	50	1.1	5.1	30	155
Tuna, bluefin, dry heat	1.6	49	—	6.3	31	184
Salmon, sockeye, dry heat	1.9	87	1.3	11.0	46	216

Fat and Cholesterol Content of Fish—*Continued*

Product (3½ Ounces, Cooked)*	Saturated Fatty Acids (Grams)	Cholesterol (Milligrams)	Omega-3 Fatty Acids (Grams)	Total Fat[1] (Grams)	Calories from Fat[2](%)	Total Calories
Anchovy, European, dry heat	2.2	—	2.1	9.7	42	210
Herring, Atlantic, dry heat	2.6	77	2.1	11.5	51	203
Eel, dry heat	3.0	161	0.7	15.0	57	236
Mackerel, Atlantic, dry heat	4.2	75	1.3	17.8	61	262
Pompano, Florida, dry heat	4.5	64	—	12.1	52	211
Crustaceans						
Lobster, northern	0.1	72	0.1	0.6	6	98
Crab, blue, moist heat	0.2	100	0.5	1.8	16	102
Shrimp, mixed species, moist heat	0.3	195	0.3	1.1	10	99
Mollusks						
Whelk, moist heat	0.1	130	—	0.8	3	275
Clam, mixed species, moist heat	0.2	67	0.3	2.0	12	148
Mussel, blue, moist heat	0.9	56	0.8	4.5	23	172
Oyster, Eastern, moist heat	1.3	109	1.0	5.0	33	137

*3½ ozs = 100 grams (approximately).

[1]Total fat = saturated fatty acids plus monounsaturated fatty acids plus polyunsaturated fatty acids.

[2]Percent calories from fat = (total fat calories divided by total calories) multiplied by 100; total fat calories = total fat (grams) multiplied by 9.

— = information not available in sources used.

Source: *Composition of Foods: Finfish and Shellfish Products—Raw * Processed * Prepared, Agriculture Handbook 8-15*. United States Department of Agriculture (in press).

Fat and Cholesterol Content of Sweets and Snacks

Product	Saturated Fatty Acids (Grams)	Cholesterol (Milligrams)	Total Fat[1] (Grams)	Calories from Fat[2](%)	Total Calories
Beverages					
Ginger ale, 12 oz.	0.0	0	0.0	0	125
Cola, regular, 12 oz.	0.0	0	0.0	0	160
Chocolate shake, 10 oz.	6.5	37	10.5	26	360
Candy (1 ounce)					
Hard candy	0.0	0	0.0	0	110
Gum drops	tr.	0	tr.	tr.	100
Fudge	2.1	1	3.0	24	115
Milk chocolate, plain	5.4	6	9.0	56	145
Cookies					
Vanilla wafers, 5 cookies, 1¾" diameter	0.9	12	3.3	32	94
Fig bars, 4 cookies, 1⅝" x 1⅝" x ⅜"	1.0	27	4.0	17	210
Chocolate brownie with icing, 1½" x 1¾" x ⅞"	1.6	14	4.0	36	100
Oatmeal cookies, 4 cookies, 2⅝" diameter	2.5	2	10.0	37	245
Chocolate chip cookies, 4 cookies, 2¼" diameter	3.9	18	11.0	54	185
Cakes and Pies					
Angel food cake, 1/12 of 10" cake	tr.	0	tr.	tr.	125
Gingerbread, 1/9 of 8" cake	1.1	1	4.0	21	175
White layer cake with white icing, 1/16 of 9" cake	2.1	3	9.0	32	260

Fat and Cholesterol Content of Sweets and Snacks—*Continued*

Product	Saturated Fatty Acids (Grams)	Cholesterol (Milligrams)	Total Fat[1] (Grams)	Calories from Fat[2](%)	Total Calories
Yellow layer cake with chocolate icing, 1/16 of 9" cake	3.0	36	8.0	31	235
Pound cake, 1/17 of loaf	3.0	64	5.0	41	110
Devil's food cake with chocolate icing, 1/16 of 9" cake	3.5	37	8.0	31	235
Lemon meringue pie, 1/6 of 9" pie	4.3	143	14.0	36	355
Apple pie, 1/6 of 9" pie	4.6	0	18.0	40	405
Cream pie, 1/6 of 9" pie	15.0	8	23.0	46	455
Snacks					
Popcorn, air-popped, 1 cup	tr.	0	tr.	tr.	30
Pretzels, stick, 2¼", 10 pretzels	tr.	0	tr.	tr.	10
Popcorn with oil and salted, 1 cup	0.5	0	3.0	49	55
Corn chips, 1 oz.	1.4	25	9.0	52	155
Potato chips, 1 oz.	2.6	0	10.1	62	147
Pudding					
Gelatin	0.0	0	0.0	0	70
Tapioca, ½ cup	2.3	15	4.0	25	145
Chocolate pudding, ½ cup	2.4	15	4.0	24	150

[1]Total fat = saturated fatty acids plus monounsaturated fatty acids plus polyunsaturated fatty acids.

[2]Percent calories from fat = (total fat calories divided by total calories) multiplied by 100; total fat calories = total fat (grams) multiplied by 9.

oz. = ounce

tr. = trace

Source: *Home and Garden Bulletin. Nutritive Value of Foods.* No. 72. United States Department of Agriculture, Human Nutrition Information Service (1986).

Fat and Cholesterol Content of Other Foods

Product	Saturated Fatty Acids (Grams)	Cholesterol (Milligrams)	Total Fat[1] (Grams)	Calories from Fat[2](%)	Total Calories
Gravies (½ cup)					
Au jus, canned	0.1	1	0.3	3	80
Turkey, canned	0.7	3	2.5	37	61
Beef, canned	1.4	4	2.8	41	62
Chicken, canned	1.7	3	6.8	65	95
Sauces (½ cup)					
Sweet and sour	tr.	0	0.1	<1	147
Barbecue	0.3	0	2.3	22	94
White	3.2	17	6.7	50	121
Cheese	4.7	26	8.6	50	154
Sour cream	8.5	45	15.1	53	255
Hollandaise	20.9	94	34.1	87	353
Bearnaise	20.9	99	34.1	88	351
Salad Dressings (1 Tablespoon)					
Russian, low calorie	0.1	1	0.7	27	23
French, low calorie	0.1	1	0.9	37	22
Italian, low calorie	0.2	1	1.5	85	16
Thousand Island, low calorie	0.2	2	1.6	59	24
Imitation mayonnaise	0.5	4	2.9	75	35
Thousand Island, regular	0.9	—	5.6	86	59
Italian, regular	1.0	—	7.1	93	69
Russian, regular	1.1	—	7.8	92	76
French, regular	1.5	—	6.4	86	67
Blue cheese	1.5	—	8.0	93	77
Mayonnaise	1.6	8	11.0	100	99
Other					
Olives, green, 4 medium	0.2	0	1.5	90	15
Nondairy creamer, powdered, 1 teaspoon	0.7	0	1.0	90	10

Fat and Cholesterol Content of Other Foods—*Continued*

Product	Saturated Fatty Acids (Grams)	Cholesterol (Milligrams)	Total Fat[1] (Grams)	Calories from Fat[2](%)	Total Calories
Avocado, Florida	5.3	0	27.0	72	340
Pizza, cheese, ⅛ of 15" diameter	4.1	56	9.0	28	290
Quiche lorraine, ⅛ of 8" diameter	23.2	285	48.0	72	600

[1]Total fat = saturated fatty acids plus monounsaturated fatty acids plus polyunsaturated fatty acids.

[2]Percent calories from fat = (total fat calories divided by total calories) multiplied by 100; total fat calories = total fat (grams) multiplied by 9.

— = information not available in sources used.

Sources: *Composition of Foods: Fats and Oils—Raw * Processed * Prepared, Agriculture Handbook 8-4*. United States Department of Agriculture, Science and Education Administration (June 1979).

*Composition of Foods: Soups, Sauces, and Gravies—Raw * Processed * Prepared, Agriculture Handbook 8-6*. United States Department of Agriculture, Science and Education Administration (February 1980).

Home and Garden Bulletin. Nutritive Value of Foods. No. 72. United States Department of Agriculture. Human Nutrition Information Service (1986).

Glossary

Adipose. The scientific term for fat tissue or body fat.

Antioxidant. Any one of a large group of substances (natural or synthetic) whose presence slows down the deterioration caused by oxygen or other substances.

Bile acids. Bile acids are emulsifying agents (detergents) made from cholesterol in the liver and stored in the gallbladder. They break up fat into smaller droplets, exposing a larger surface area of the fats to the action of fat-digesting enzymes, which increase fat digestion.

Cholesterol. A complex fatty substance which can be made in the body or supplied through foods of animal origin. It has many important functions in the body; however, excess cholesterol may be deposited in artery linings.

Choline. A vitamin involved in nerve function and the metabolism of fats. It is found in ample quantities in lecithin (phosphatidyl choline).

Cold pressed. A commonly misused term which implies that an oil has been extracted without the use of chemical solvents.

Eicosapentaenoic acid. The substance from which the body makes the series 3 prostaglandins. It is found in high quantities in cold-water fish and marine animals.

Emulsify. To break up into smaller drops by the actions of detergents.

Enzyme. A protein produced by the body to facilitate (catalyze) particular chemical reactions, but which itself is unchanged by the reaction.

Essential fatty acid. Either of two fatty acids, linoleic acid or linolenic acid, that the body requires and cannot make from other substances. EFAs must be supplied by food.

Evening primrose. A plant whose seeds contain the essential linoleic acid.

Fat. Three fatty acids hooked to a glycerol molecule in an ester linkage. In common usage, it refers to those substances that fit the above description, and are hard at room temperature because they contain mostly saturated fatty acids.

Fatty acid. A carbon chain having an organic acid group at one end, with hydrogens attached to the rest of the carbon atoms in the chain.

Fatty degeneration. Fatty deposits commonly found in the arteries, around tumors, and in the liver and other internal organs that interfere with normal biological functions.

Fiber. Any of several indigestible complex carbohydrates that form the "roughage" of plant material. Fiber aids in bowel regularity, helps to stabilize blood sugar, and aids in the elimination of cholesterol and bile acids from the body.

Free radical. A molecule or molecular fragment with a single or unpaired electron. Since it is seeking to be paired, this fragment steals electrons from other pairs. Although free radical reactions generally occur in normal biological processes, they can pose a danger when they are involved in a chain reaction.

Free radical chain reaction. An uncontrolled free radical reaction. These reactions are generally damaging to biological processes.

Gamma linolenic acid. A substance found in mother's milk and evening primrose oil. It is made from the essential linoleic acid by healthy cells.

HDL. *See* High-density lipoprotein.

High-density lipoprotein. A substance found in the bloodstream that carries fats and cholesterol. It is the "good" type of cholesterol, which returns excess cholesterol from the cells to the liver, where it is changed into bile acids that enter into the intestine to aid in fat digestion and are then excreted by the body.

Hydrogenation. A commercial process that turns oils into fats by destroying the double bonds in the fatty acids and saturating the carbon atoms with hydrogen.

LDL. *See* Low-density lipoprotein.

Lecithin. A nutritious substance consisting of glycerol, fatty acids, phosphate groups, and choline. Soybeans and egg yolks are a good source of lecithin, which contains both essential fatty acids.

Linoleic acid. One of the two essential fatty acids. It is required for life, and since the body cannot make it, it must be obtained from food. The body makes several other important substances from it.

Linolenic acid. One of the two essential fatty acids. It is extremely sensitive to oxygen, light, and high temperatures, all of which can destroy it. Its absence from the diet is fatal. Deficiency is linked to degenerative disease.

Lipid. The chemist's collective name for fats, oils, and other fatty substances.

Lipoprotein. Transport vehicles for fats and cholesterol in the blood and lymph. Generally speaking, fatty substances (oils, fats, phosphatides, and cholesterol) associated with protein materials.

Low-density lipoprotein. Known as the "bad" type of cholesterol, this substance carries excess cholesterol and deposits it along the arterial walls.

Oil. A liquid fat. The shorter the fatty acid chains (or the more double bonds present in them), the more liquid the oil.

Oxidize. The addition of oxygen, subtraction of hydrogen, or addition of electrons to a substance. Oxidation is usually accompanied by a release of energy.

Partially hydrogenated. An oil in which most of the double bonds have been destroyed by the addition, under pressure and high temperature, of hydrogen to the fatty acid molecules. The result is a semi-solid fat. Many chemical changes take place in the fatty acid molecules during this process.

Phosphatide. Also called a phospholipid. A class of fatty compounds found in the membranes. Lecithin is the most well known of the phosphatides. Phosphatides consist of two fatty acid molecules, a glycerol molecule, a phosphate group, and some other groups hooked to the phosphate.

Polyunsaturated. A fatty acid that contains more than one double bond between carbon atoms in its chain. The term includes both natural, healthful fatty acids and unnatural, detrimental ones.

Prostaglandin. A fatty acid with hormonelike functions in the regulation of cell activity. About thirty different prostaglandins are known. These fatty acids are partially oxidized, and are controlled by enzymes made in the body for just this purpose.

Saturated fatty acid. A fatty acid with every possible position on the carbon atoms taken up by hydrogen atoms and no double bonds in the carbon chain.

Short-chain fatty acid. A fatty acid with ten or less carbon atoms in its chain.

Triglyceride. A molecule of fat or oil consisting of three fatty acid molecules hooked to glycerol.

Unsaturated fatty acid. A fatty acid with one or more double bonds between carbons in its chain.

Vitamin E. A natural antioxidant and essential vitamin that is found in seeds containing oil and required by the body to prevent the destruction of membrane fatty acids by oxidation.

References

CHAPTER 2

Deuel, H.J., Jr. *The Lipids: Their Chemistry*. New York: Interscience Publishers, 1951.

Williams, Sue Rodwell. *Nutrition and Diet Therapy*. St. Louis: C.V. Mosy and Company, 1969.

CHAPTER 3

Brody, Jane E. "It's Not Just Calories, It's Their Source," *The New York Times*. 12 July 1988, sec. C, p. 3.

MacNeil, Karen. "Diet Soft Drinks: Too Good to Be True?" *The New York Times*. 4 February 1987, sec. C, p. 3.

"Research Lifts Blame From Many of the Obese," *The New York Times*, 24 March 1987, sec. C, p. 1.

"Sad News for Dieters," *Working Together Bulletin*. Dartnell Corporation, 1986.

CHAPTER 5

"Early Detection, Treatment and Low Fat Diet Can Help Prevent Adult Hearing Loss," *The New York Times*, 2 October 1985.

Kolata, Gina. "New Theory Explains How Cholesterol Threatens the Heart," *The New York Times*, 25 October 1988.

Stukane, Eileen. "Health Eating," *Food & Wine Magazine*, May 1988, p. 124.

CHAPTER 7

"Safety Factors to Consider," *The New York Times*, 27 July 1983, sec. C., p. 8.

Stukane, Eileen. "Health Eating," *Food & Wine Magazine*, May 1988, p. 124.

About the Author

Lewis Harrison is a highly respected researcher, writer, teacher, and consultant in the areas of nutrition, natural healing, and creative personal development. As director of the Health Associates organization in the late 1970s, Lewis developed one of the most comprehensive programs in the world for gathering data on contemporary health care.

Lewis has been a member of the prestigious New York Academy of Sciences and a feature editor for a medical journal. He has served as a post-graduate instructor at the Swedish Institute in New York City.

Lewis's work has been cited in numerous articles and magazines. He has appeared on a host of radio and television talk shows throughout the United States. Lewis has also been listed in the International Directory of Distinguished Leadership.

In addition to his past position as vice-president of the New York chapter of the American Massage Therapy Association (AMTA), Lewis has been on the advisory board of the AMTA journal. Besides writing many articles for various magazines and periodicals over the last fifteen years, he is the author of two other successful health-related titles, *Massageworks*, which he co-authored, and *Helping Yourself With Natural Healing*.

Lewis Harrison currently resides in New York City. To receive more information or a free copy of Lewis Harrison's Nutrition Newsletter, write to Lewis Harrison, Box 315, Ansonia Station, New York, New York 10023.

Index